Human–Computer Interface Technologies for the Motor Impaired

REHABILITATION SCIENCE IN PRACTICE SERIES

Series Editors

Marcia J. Scherer, Ph.D.

President
Institute for Matching Person and Technology

Professor
Physical Medicine & Rehabilitation University of Rochester Medical Center

Dave Muller, Ph.D.

Executive
Suffolk New College

Editor-in-Chief
Disability and Rehabilitation

Founding Editor
Aphasiology

Published Titles

Ambient Assisted Living, *Nuno M. Garcia and Joel J.P.C. Rodrigues*

Assistive Technology Assessment Handbook, *edited by Stefano Federici and Marcia J. Scherer*

Assistive Technology for Blindness and Low Vision, *Roberto Manduchi and Sri Kurniawan*

Computer Access for People with Disabilities: A Human Factors Approach,
     Richard C. Simpson

Computer Systems Experiences of Users with and Without Disabilities: An Evaluation Guide
     for Professionals, *Simone Borsci, Maria Laura Mele, Masaaki Kurosu, and Stefano Federici*

Devices for Mobility and Manipulation for People with Reduced Abilities,
     Teodiano Bastos-Filho, Dinesh Kumar, and Sridhar Poosapadi Arjunan

Human–Computer Interface Technologies for the Motor Impaired,
     edited by Dinesh K. Kumar and Sridhar Poosapadi Arjunan

Multiple Sclerosis Rehabilitation: From Impairment to Participation,
     edited by Marcia Finlayson

Neuroprosthetics: Principles and Applications, *edited by Justin Sanchez*

Paediatric Rehabilitation Engineering: From Disability to Possibility, *edited by Tom Chau
     and Jillian Fairley*

Quality of Life Technology Handbook, *Richard Schultz*

Rehabilitation: A Post-critical Approach, *edited by Barbara E. Gibson*

Rehabilitation Goal Setting: Theory, Practice and Evidence, *edited by Richard J. Siegert
     and William M. M. Levack*

Rethinking Rehabilitation: Theory and Practice, *edited by Kathryn McPherson,
     Barbara E. Gibson, and Alain Leplège*

Human–Computer Interface Technologies for the Motor Impaired

Dinesh K. Kumar
RMIT University, Melbourne, Victoria, Australia

Sridhar Poosapadi Arjunan
Biomedical Engineering, School of EE, RMIT University, Melbourne

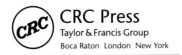

CRC Press
Taylor & Francis Group
Boca Raton London New York

CRC Press is an imprint of the
Taylor & Francis Group, an **informa** business

CRC Press
Taylor & Francis Group
6000 Broken Sound Parkway NW, Suite 300
Boca Raton, FL 33487-2742

© 2016 by Taylor & Francis Group, LLC
CRC Press is an imprint of Taylor & Francis Group, an Informa business

No claim to original U.S. Government works

Printed on acid-free paper
Version Date: 20150811

International Standard Book Number-13: 978-1-4822-6266-7 (Hardback)

Visit the Taylor & Francis Web site at
http://www.taylorandfrancis.com

and the CRC Press Web site at
http://www.crcpress.com

Contents

8 Video-based eye tracking   117

9 Speech for controlling computers   135

List of Figures

List of Tables

Preface

It all began when I received a call from one lady one sunny afternoon in Melbourne. She introduced herself as a "Granny from the bush" and asked me to help her identify technologies that her grandson could use for controlling his computer games. The boy suffered muscle wasting of the upper limb and was unable to perform the actions, and she was keen for him to play these games so that he will make friends and socialize. I do not know how she got my name or telephone number, or why she thought that I would and could help her, but this phone call made me think. I ended up spending many of my hours searching for the relevant information. It was quite evident that she had attempted to search things by herself but was unable to obtain suitable information. The information was either too technical or too much of sales pitch, and there was no place where she could compare the different technologies.

Different from the aforementioned telecon, I had a meeting with nurses working with people requiring continuing assistance and realized that the problem was not confined to an elderly grandmother but was also felt by qualified nurses. Thanks to the all-present Internet, and various search engines, they were aware that there were numbers of sources of information. However, they felt that these are either "hard sell" or too technical, and took a lot of their time. I realized that although there were large numbers of very good journals reporting the research and development work in the field, and there were many universities that now have a separate department for conducting research in developing computer interfaces, there was no book that suitably covered the topic. There was no book or platform that could be useful for scientists, engineers, clinicians, and laypeople alike. There was no platform that encourages the interaction between these groups of people. This established my purpose of writing this book.

When I began writing this book, I was expecting that I will be able to obtain the required information from various papers and technical reports and consolidate it. However, I soon realized that I had a bigger project on my hands than simply collecting the works of others. I realized that all research papers, while working in this multidisciplinary field, were very narrowly focused and that was the reason why the grandmother required to call me for help or the nurses would simply direct their patients to a shop. At this stage, I invited Dr. Sridhar Arjunan to join the team and we began writing this book.

As researchers, we have published extensively and similar to most research papers, our papers target a specialized audience who knows the specific field extensively. While human–computer interfaces (HCIs) for people with disabilities require a multidisciplinary approach, most scientific papers tend to focus on very specific topics. This is essential for research in the field, but these papers become exclusive. Thus, papers discussing the hardware, the software, clinical relevance, and rehabilitation aspects appear to be highly focused, and often may not find the audience in the other disciplines. This gave me the biggest challenge: to write the outcomes of the research work of our team and of many others reported in literature, but suitable for researchers, engineers, clinicians, and laypeople. I decided to focus the book on ensuring that it is inclusive and suitable for being understood by all the stakeholders, thereby encouraging greater dialogue.

For the research audience, we have provided sufficient details to encourage cross-discipline dialogue between different fields of research. We also expect that this will encourage a dialogue between the researchers and other stakeholders and help the outcome of their research to enhance customer and patient focus.

For our engineering readers, we anticipate that this book will provide them with better understanding of the science behind the works, and user requirements of the clinicians and end users. This would lead to improved HCI devices that are more suited for the users and reduce the negative impact of disabilities in our society. We anticipate that this would also lead to greater participation by technology entrepreneurs and thus leading to enhanced competition and more options for the customers.

For our clinical-focused readers, this book will lead to their better understanding of the technology. They will be in a stronger position to guide their patients and help the patients understand the range of possibilities and limitations. We also hope that this will encourage them to participate in the dialogue with researchers and scientists to identify the strengths and limitations of the various technologies, and thus give the very important feedback to the researchers, developers, and engineers.

And finally we anticipate that this book will greatly benefit the end users and their carers. It will provide the information of many of the devices and technologies such that the users can assess these from the view point of their personal requirements. Each of us is different, and such information will enable the end users to select what is best for them, without the bias that is presented by sales pitches of commercial organizations. Such knowledge will also enable them to identify the improvements that they require, and thus participate in a dialogue with government bodies, companies, and scientists. This book should provide them the strength to participate in the future dialogues and in recommending further research and improvements.

We also anticipate that this book would be useful for people developing devices such as computer games or machine consoles. The computer games market is in excess of $100 billion and with an estimated 500 million regular users, there are many opportunities for the industry to absorb advanced human–computer interface devices. This can be very useful for the HCI researchers and industry because it will lead to greater funding opportunity and thus innovation.

We are hopeful that this book is the start of a dialogue and leads to an improved interaction between different stakeholders of computer interfaces.

Professor Dinesh K. Kumar

Acknowledgment

We would like to thank the following researchers for their work, contribution, and involvement in the research studies mentioned in this book:

Professor Teodiano Bastos, Professor Hirokazu Shimada, Dr. Eric Poole, Dr. Arun Sharma, Dr. Sanjay Kumar, Dr. Wai Chee Yau, Dr. Vijay Pal Singh, Dr. Behzad Aliahmad, and Linglong Li.

Authors

Dinesh K. Kumar received a BTech from IIT Madras and a PhD in biomedical engineering from IIT Delhi and AIIMS, Delhi. He is a professor and leader of biomedical engineering at RMIT University, Melbourne, Australia. He has published more than 330 refereed papers in the field, and his interests include muscle control, affordable diagnostics, and human–computer interface. He is editor of multiple journals and chairs a range of conferences related to biomedical engineering. He enjoys walking in nature in his spare time.

Sridhar Poosapadi Arjunan received a BEng in electronics and communication from the University of Madras, India; MEng in communication systems from Madurai Kamaraj University, India; and earned a PhD in biomedical signal processing from RMIT University, Melbourne, Australia. He is currently a postdoctoral research fellow with Biosignals Lab at RMIT University. He is a recipient of the RMIT SECE Research Scholarship, CASS Australian Early Career Researcher grant, and Australia-India ECR fellowship. His major research interests include biomedical signal processing, rehabilitation study, fractal theory, and human–computer interface applications.

CHAPTER ONE

Introduction

Abstract

Technology has resulted in our ability to control machines for improving our lives. However, large number of people around the world are unable to use the conventional machine interface devices due to injury, disease, or simply weakness due to aging. This chapter introduces the reader to the requirement and the fundamental concept of human–computer interface (HCI) and lists the different modalities that are available. The different applications of each modality have been discussed and it introduces the reader to the next nine chapters.

1.1 Introduction: Human–computer interface for people with disabilities

It is commonly said that our ability to build machines is what differentiates us from other animals, because machines provide us with the ability to perform actions that would have been otherwise impossible. We are able to move mountains, dig tunnels, and move places using the machines that we have developed over the past centuries. The famous statement that is attributed to Archimedes: "Give me a lever long enough and a fulcrum on which to place it, and I shall move the world." Thus, machines are devices that allow us to outdo the abilities of our bodies.

Machines have broken the barriers that were based on physical abilities and people of all sizes, age, and irrespective of gender are able to perform tasks that they would earlier not have been able to do. Irrespective of the size of the person, we are able to drive large trucks and even mining equipment, and control computers without requiring us to be experts in computers. All these have been possible because of interfaces that enable humans to control machines.

The ability to control machines is an essential part of being the modern human and controlling machines is a necessary part of our lives. The machines and machine control systems have often been designed for the majority of the users. Thus, our current systems are based on the use of devices such as levers, wheels, keyboards, and mouse that we are able to control nearly all the equipment that is required for modern living and industry. These devices have, in general, broken the barriers for women to enter professions that were until recently reserved for men. With the availability of powered tools, industries such as building and construction, which were until recently the bastion for young men, are now open to people of both genders and all sizes.

The availability of powered technologies has also enabled the ability of people of both genders and of range of age to participate actively in activities such as defense and shipping. However, although the development has broken many barriers, these technologies have largely been developed for the majority of people, and there is an assumption that the users have dexterity of their hands, and are able to receive sensory feedback such as visual, pressure, and movement. Overcoming this shortcoming is the focus of large number of companies and research teams around the world, and comes under the generic umbrella of HCI for people with disabilities.

1.2 Background

Medical advances have enhanced our longevity and we are living longer than ever before in history. Modern medicine has also improved the likelihood for the survival of many people who have suffered neuromuscular or skeletal injuries. Our society has a significant number of people who are weak due to aging, or have lost their ability to perform number of actions due to disease or injury. Thus, we have a large number of people who require assistive technologies to perform functions that the majority of the population would do routinely.

Assistive technologies range from mobility devices such as wheelchairs, artificial hands, communication devices, and control interfaces to manage the surroundings. These devices range in complexity based on the level of support required by the patients. Loss of mobility is the single largest cause of major disability and may be caused due to number of reasons such as trauma or disease. The global estimate of people who suffer and survive spinal cord injury (SCI) every year is 22 people per million inhabitants or more than 130,000 people each year worldwide [1]. In Australia, it has been estimated that there are 241 SCI injuries per annum, which correspond to 13.2 people/million inhabitants. A majority of these patients become dependent on a wheelchair for their entire lives. However, the number of users of wheelchairs is significantly higher than the people who have suffered an SCI.

With scientific advancement, there is increased awareness and this has resulted in the changes of the aspirations and requirements by patients who have suffered disabilities, by the elderly, and the society in general. People like to live independently and neither be bound to their beds or hospitals, nor be dependent on their carer to take them out or to communicate with the rest of the world.

There is also the cost basis, because the healthcare system is unable to support the need for caring for the burgeoning number of people who require assistance in performing their regular tasks. Healthcare is unable to support such a large number of people in assistive living conditions due to the cost of caring and nursing. Technology that can facilitate independent living for the disabled or the elderly is thus a win-win situation. This has resulted in greater demands for technologies that can assist people in leading independent lives.

Powered devices and the Internet are now in all facets of our lives, and have provided the means for removing the barriers between genders in access to activities and tasks that were earlier required a specific body size and type. This has also facilitated the disabled to lead independent lives and one significant example is the use of powered wheelchairs and scooters that allow the disabled and the elderly travel without a carer having to wheel them around. The Internet allows people to experience the world or to communicate with the rest of the world without having to move out of their rooms. However, the success of these requires the user to appropriately interface with these devices, and thus the need for a suitable computer interface. Such interface devices are referred to as HCI for the disabled people.

1.3 History

Machines provide users with the ability to perform tasks that they would otherwise be unable to comfortably perform. One of the earliest machines incorporated the mechanical concepts of the levers and wheels. To control these devices required the users to have strength and precision, and the early mechanisms to control machines required mechanical levers and springs, which typically required the strength and precision of the user. With technical advancements in areas such as fluidics, these got transformed to the use of hydraulics, and with advancements in the electrical engineering, the users were able to control machines with the help of electrical switches.

Electronics opened a new era that allowed the person to control devices using very small devices that did not require big wires and high voltages, and thus were suitable even for children to use. Developments in the area of sensors furthered the ability of people to remotely sense and monitor machines, and control the equipment from a safe and comfortable location. However, it is the recent developments in the areas of wireless electronics, computers, and biomedical engineering that have taken the machine control to new heights.

Recent developments in the field of computers have facilitated the use of computerized control systems, and we are able to control nearly all machines to the required precision. Thus, there is no longer the necessity of the person to understand the method for controlling a machine or a device, because the computers have been programmed to do this. The users are provided with suitable interfaces such as a screen and devices such as keyboard or mouse by which they can command the machine. Thus, to control a large machine does not require the user to be a muscular person and a small-build person can do this as easily.

The revolution in the field of wireless technologies has facilitated the use sensing of the conditions and actuating a machine from anywhere. The control of the robotic devices sent to Mars has shown that this can be achieved from even another planet. With the availability of mobile phones, the Internet, and wireless technologies, we can control any device from literally anywhere in the world. This has also provided the ability of remote monitoring of devices and situations. This provides the person to control the machines from their offices rather than having to be in places that are uncomfortable and remote.

Another significant contributor to our ability to control and communicate with remote machines is the advancement in signal processing and classification. There has been large progress in the area of signal processing and classification. Advanced signal processing has resulted in the development of speech analysis techniques that recognize the speech and the speaker. Thus, the voice recording can be used to obtain what the user said, and the speech of the user can be converted to text. This is now incorporated in most computers, tablets, and mobile phones. Thus, computer-based systems can be controlled by spoken commands, and speech-based typing systems are now available. This is a major step in machine control and communication systems because it allows people to control devices without using their hands, or "hands-free" mode.

Biomedical engineering is human centric and has advanced very significantly over the past 50 years. Biomedical engineering and science has discovered the details of the functioning of the brain, the neural system, and muscle control. These advancements have provided a mechanism for users to give commands directly from their brain or nerves, without having to make any movement. This has taken the concept of machine control to a new level, where the user is able to command or communicate with only their thoughts, and without having to make any movement of their limbs, or even without needing to verbalize their commands.

Many SCI patients require lifelong care, and this is a significant cost to the healthcare system. In less affluent nations, the number is higher, and because of the lack of resources, the suffering of these people is greater. With the growth of technology and social awareness, society is not comfortable in accepting that disabled people are unable to control machines, communicate, or be entertained. Although people with disabilities were earlier expected to accept the fate of their inabilities, disabled people now are demanding greater independence. Thus, over the years, there has been growth in the number of devices and technologies that they can use to control machines and computers even if they lack dexterity of their hands, or strength in their limbs or even if they lack the ability to perform functions such as speaking and moving their eyes. For people who have lost all motor control or sensory capabilities, there are interfaces that are directly commanded by their brain activity and based on their thoughts.

1.4 Future of HCI

HCI is a field that is developing at a very rapid pace. It is identified as an independent field of research, and there are number of journals and conferences that are dedicated to this field of research. Whereas earlier work was to facilitate the disabled people, help them regain some of their freedom, and give them independence in performing their daily activities, HCI is now significantly superior and better. It provides the elderly and the weak with the ability to lead their lives independently, for people with lost hearing to hear, and helps the blind to see again. HCI also facilitates the disabled to be entertained and they can use it to browse the Web, listen to music, communicate, and watch movies. HCI is not limited to the people with reduced abilities but is also being adapted by able-bodied people to play computer games or participate in immersive virtual reality. The technology has also been adapted for number of defense applications and is now being used for controlling vehicles and weapons.

HCI is now not limited to engineering laboratories but is also an integral part of modern medicine. The field provides the ability for helping hearing-impaired individuals, and more recently progress is being made for helping blind people to see again. HCI is now used by disabled people for a number of applications such as to type without a keyboard on their computer, communicate with others, and control their wheelchairs. However, current systems have limitations and often suffer from poor reliability and limited degrees of freedom. The focus of research in number of teams is to improve the reliability, give greater freedom to the user, and make the interface more natural for the user. With advancement in surgical procedures, better understanding of the human brain, wireless technologies, and smaller and smarter electronic devices, implanted systems are now being considered as one of the major options of the future. There is also greater focus on the use of systems that learn and configure to the user using techniques such as intelligent agents and other methods.

The progress in this field is very rapid, and there is no crystal ball that can predict the future. However, it is very evident that technologies that provide the near-natural and seamless commanding and sensing abilities to disabled users are desired. A reasonable statement is that the future will include both invasive and noninvasive techniques and will not be limited to a single modality. With the advancement in computational strengths and widespread networking capabilities, it is conceivable that the future technologies would be user focused and dedicated to each user, based on their personal conditions and requirements.

1.5 Layout of the book

This book describes a range of HCI technologies. These range from simple modification of the current devices such as the modified computer mouse and joystick, to a brain–computer interface (BCI) that uses the electrical recording of the brain activity of the user. Although no single book can describe each device that has been developed and reported in literature, this book describes the fundamentals that would be the basis for most devices.

Each chapter in this book describes a specific technology and lists some of the major strengths and shortcomings. The fundamentals associated with the generic technology have been described and a specific example of the technology has been detailed. Ongoing research in the field has been discussed and suitable literature has been reviewed. The intent is to provide the user with comprehensive knowledge of the technology and its applications. Readers who are specifically looking for details have been provided with a list of some of the major publications in the field. In most cases, the details of the mathematical rigor associated with the technique are not given in this book, but suitable references have been provided.

Chapter 2 examines interface devices based on mechanical sensors. This chapter provides the details of mechanical sensors that are used as interface to control a computer or a screen for aged and disabled people. Incorporating these technologies for working systems, different options, applications, and the limitations are also discussed.

Chapter 3 describes the BCI using brain waves recorded by noninvasive electrodes to recognize the command from the user. This chapter introduces the fundamentals of brain waves, the method for recording the electroencephalogram, and some methods for the analysis. The current technologies and implementation are described, with the possible applications, user requirements, and limitations.

Chapter 4 discusses evoked potential-based techniques for recognizing the commands from the user. After discussing the concept of evoked potential-based BCI, the method for recording and analyzing the signals are explained. The applications and limitations of the technique are identified. One example of the implementation of steady-state visual-evoked potential, along with the applications, user requirements, and limitations are described.

Chapter 5 describes the myoelectric interface for controlling devices such as the prosthetic/robotic hand. This chapter introduces the technology of recording myoelectric signals, some of the methods used to analyze the signals, and the parameters for the system. The implementation of one myoelectric-based HCI is described in detail. This chapter also provides information regarding the limitations and challenges that exist due to the gross nature of the signal, presence of cross talk, noise, and other factors that are required to be overcome in the future.

Chapter 6 discusses the technologies for recognizing hand gestures and movements from videos and the challenges associated with the real-time implementations. Recognition of commands from the video of the user has the advantage because these are nonintrusive. HCI based on the video has been extensively improved in recent years in gaming applications. This chapter describes some of the applications of these video-based systems for disabled people.

Chapter 7 describes an HCI system based on the electrooculogram signal, which is the electrical potential corresponding to the eye gaze and recorded from around the eyes. This chapter describes the techniques to record and analyze the electrooculogram for controlling a computer mouse or a machine, and one implementation is described in detail. Applications and limitations of these techniques are also discussed.

Chapter 8 follows from Chapters 6 and 7, and describes the technology of tracking the eye gaze using video technology. In this chapter, a comparison is provided between video and bioelectric signal-based eye gaze recognition. An implementation of the technology has been described. The applications and shortcomings of these technologies, and future directions are discussed.

Chapter 9 provides the fundamentals of voice recognition technologies for computer and machine control applications. This chapter describes the signal analysis and classification algorithms, and provides a comparison between the different methods. The applications and limitations are discussed and future directions identified.

Chapter 10 examines a secure and voiceless method for the recognition of speech-based commands using video of lip movement. The major drawback with the use of sound for computer control such as for Internet access is that the commands are audible to other people in the vicinity and the user does not enjoy the privacy. This chapter discusses the possible applications and limitations of the technology, and the current research activity that is taking place in this field.

Reference

1. ICCP, International Campaign for Cures of Spinal Cord Injury Paralysis. Available at: http://www.campaignforcure.org. Accessed July 6, 2015.

CHAPTER TWO

Human–computer interface

Mechanical sensors

Abstract

The computer mouse, smart screen, and joystick are some of the mechanical devices that are used by most people to control a computer or other similar devices. However, a significant number of people with disabilities or due to weaknesses, or who are in special circumstances are unable to use such devices. A number of mechanical-based interfaces are now available that facilitate such users to control machines and computers. One example is the smart glove, which is a technology that has embedded mechanical sensors that can identify the intended command of the user. This chapter describes these technologies, and discusses the different options, applications, and the limitations.

2.1 Introduction

The joystick, computer mouse, or tablet screen are routinely used to control computerized equipment and are now an essential part of our modern lives. However, people in special conditions may be unable to perform such actions and they need to control the machine such as a computer or a robotic device with other options and not these commonly available devices. This may be because these people are in special situations such as defense personnel or for those who lack fine control of the hand that provides the required dexterity or for applications such as computer games [1]. Over the years, numerous different modalities have been developed to address these needs. This chapter describes some of these options.

A number of devices that sense the user commands mechanically have been developed and are suited for people who are unable to use commonly available devices such as the computer mouse [2]. While some of these are modifications of the existing devices, there are other devices that have been specifically developed for people with special needs. All devices that use mechanical sensing require movement by the user and are suitable for people who have the appropriate level of motor activity, though they may not have the dexterity that is demonstrated by able-bodied counterparts. These sensors are described in the following sections.

2.2 Modified devices

For many applications, appropriate modification of the computer interface provides suitable outcomes. Some of the examples are the modification of the computer mouse and joystick, trackball, and computer tablet. These are described in the following sections.

2.2.1 Mouse or joystick

For a number of applications, the simple modification of the mouse or joystick may be sufficient to facilitate the user with special needs to use a computer or similar device, and many of these products are commonly available [3,4]. There are many choices for the modified mouse, and customized joysticks also provide an alternate control (Figure 2.1). Some of the other devices that have been used are steering wheels, thumb mouse, trackball, foot-ball trackball, extra-large joysticks, and mouse with controllable friction. Although these products are very useful in helping people who are unable to use the computer mouse or keyboard, often these are not sufficient for providing the users with easy and robust control. There are a number of devices and software solutions that have been developed especially for helping people with special needs.

2.2.2 Tracking ball

Trackball (or tracking ball) is a device that is used to point, and can be used for moving the computer cursor or similar applications [3]. It consists of a ball located in a socket that has sensors that detect the rotation of the ball about two axes. It can be considered as an upside-down ball-based mouse, with a protruding

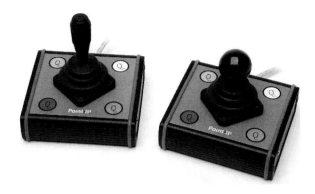

FIGURE 2.1 Example of a modified joystick. (From Unique Perspectives Ltd., Ireland. With permission.)

ball that is exposed for the user. The size of this ball can be selected based on the applications and user capability. Whereas balls of the size of 50 mm may be used for being controlled by the thumb, fingers, or the palm of the hand, larger balls are required for foot control.

The advantage of using the trackball is that there is no limit to the movement. Whereas the mouse requires a flat surface or a mouse pad, and it is effective only within the region of the surface, the trackball does not have such limitations. Further, whereas a mouse has to be gripped and positioned, the user for the trackball has to move the ball in the desired direction. Trackballs can be made with different materials, though most are made from rubber or glass. Some of these have switches located separately, although most of them will have switches placed on the plate next located with it.

Trackballs are used in many fields and by fully able-bodied people besides the people with physical disabilities. Some computer-aided design (CAD) workstations use large trackballs for improved precision, and small trackballs are sometimes used for portable computers to save keypad space.

2.2.3 Modified computer display or digital tablet

A digital tablet is touch sensitive and allows the user to slide the finger on a flat tablet. It is similar to the computer mouse pad, and the user is able to give the commands for controlling the wheelchair using this. It has the advantage that it is inexpensive and can easily replace the joystick with minimal alterations to the wheelchair controller. Wheelesley, a robotic wheelchair system developed by MIT [5], used switches on a panel onboard to choose among different high-level movement commands such as forward, left, right, stop, or drive backward, and can also be maneuvered with an eye-tracking interface.

Tablets are commonly used for users to control computers and associated machines. These are touch, or pressure sensitive, and detect the location of the contact with the user, either using the finger or a stylus. These have often been integrated with the display screens; displays such as active screens are now commonly used for interacting with computers and managing machines [6]. However, some people lack the precision or speed to sufficiently control their hands and fingers to interact with such devices. This may be caused by disease or due to aging. This can cause them to miscommunicate or make erroneous commands, leading to frustration or even injury. To overcome these problems, a number of such devices are offering the software that allows the user to change some settings such that the interaction is suited for their needs. There are, however, specially developed software and tablets for people with special needs.

There are number of software-based options that can be used to customize the tablet or screen to the user. One software solution is the modified computer screen where the regular keys are replaced by a specific set of icons that are useful for the user. Although this reduces the flexibility of the keyboard, the customizing provides the user with reliability that allows them to function safely. This provides the safety to the user, who may otherwise miscommunicate due to the inability to have fine control of the interface which has large number of keys and other options.

2.2.4 Special purpose interface devices

Modifications of existing devices are only effective for people who have significant movement of the hand or the foot. However, number of people may not have sufficient control of their hands or feet and are unable to use these devices, even after modification. For such cases, specialized devices have been developed. Some of these are head movements, blow and suck (also named "sip and puff switch"), and smart glove. These are described in the next sections.

2.2.4.1 Head movement   People who are unable to use their hands or feet, but have the movement of their neck can interface with computerized devices or give commands using the movement of the head [7]. Suitable sensors that can measure the movement of the head can be employed. The choice of the sensor is dependent on a number of factors such as the sensitivity and specificity for the user. It is important that the user does not have to make large and awkward head movements, and it is essential that unintended movement of the head are not identified by the system as commands [8]. Other factors that need to be considered are the reliability, convenience, and the aesthetics.

Although there are number of options, the purpose of the sensors is to identify the intended head movement. This can be achieved using the inertial measurement unit (IMU), angle sensors, or stretch sensors. These are described in later sections.

2.2.4.2 Blow and suck

One of the simplest yet effective means for control or communication is based on the ability of the user to control their breathing. This could be an alternate for people who do not have sufficient control of their neck, or it could be combined with other modalities to develop a hybrid system.

Blow or suck (also called sip and puff switch) can be used to command the wheelchair for users with ability of blowing and sucking a straw [9]. In this modality, a pressure sensor, installed into a straw, allows users either choosing icons for communication or movement commands of the wheelchair.

The fundamental design of these devices includes a tubing or air-straws fitted with sensors that identify the push and pull of the air. Typically, the device has two sensors: one sensor to monitor the push or air movement associated with the blowing action; and the other sensor is for detecting the pull, or the movement of air associated with the suck action. Devices that monitor the speed of airflow have also been considered because such a system will offer greater degrees of freedom, however, these are not commonly used due to the inability of the target users to effectively control the rate of air flow.

2.2.4.3 Smart glove

People with reduced motor ability or people working in high-risk conditions can benefit from gloves that can sense the detailed movement of the hand and convey this to the computer or the robotic device. Such a glove can be useful for obtaining the command of the user to control robotic devices or computer cursor [10]. These gloves can also be used for other applications such as computer games and defense technology.

The smart glove is an integration of multiple sensors that are embedded in a glove that is worn by the user. These sensors detect the hand movement such as individual finger flexion, wrist flexion, and rotation. Such a glove has the advantage that it fits directly on the hand of the user and allows the user the natural connectivity with the devices to be controlled. Some of these gloves may also contain feedback modality where the factors such as force or pressure may be sensed on the robotic device end and feedback provided to the user. The feedback may typically be in the form of vibration and often located in the palm region of the glove.

2.3 Sensors

Mechanical HCI devices require the translation of movement or force to electrical signals that are the input to the computerized device. There are a number of options for such sensing, including measure of position, acceleration, stretch, or rotation. One common factor in the sensing is the need for these sensors to be lightweight and nonintrusive. It is also important that these sensors are low powered and do not require number of wires.

An example of a position sensor is the inertial measurement units, and angles can be sensed using goniometers. Stretchable inductive coils or stretchable resistances are suitable for measuring the change in length, and load cells are examples of force sensors. Each of these sensors is described in the next sections.

2.3.1 Inertial measurement unit

An inertial measurement unit, or IMU, is an electronic device that measures and reports velocity, orientation, and gravitational forces, using a combination of accelerometers and gyroscopes, sometimes also magnetometers. IMUs are used for a number of applications including aviation and defense. These are generally lightweight, can be integrated with a global positioning system (GPS), and can measure the movement in terms of acceleration. Integration with wireless technologies such as Bluetooth allows the device to be used without cumbersome wires. Recent advancements in microdevices has resulted in making these devices lightweight and inexpensive, and thus suitable for assistive technology applications [11].

IMUs allow the integration of different techniques that can be combined to identify the motion and actions of the user. Although advanced applications can be used to identify the position and movement, and relative movement when multiple units are used, these in general are more complex and require sophisticated algorithms and software. However, recent advancements have made these more affordable, and it is but a matter of time when it may be suitable for monitoring the movement of the limbs of the user, or other body movement such as the head.

For applications such as controlling the movement of a cursor on the computer screen or the movement of the wheelchair, a relatively simpler approach is suitable. In such applications, a sensor may be embedded on the cap of the user, and the average inclination of the head is used to identify the direction of the head inclination: forward, backward, left, or right. These four directions are used to provide command of the wheelchair or a computer cursor on the screen. There may be a number of options for the sensor, such as the use of a three-dimensional (3D) accelerometer, tilt sensors, and IMU.

The head inclination angles are computed based on the associated gravitational accelerations [12]. Two independent angles are determined to obtain the head movement: α and γ angles, where α is the forward head inclination and is related to linear velocity of the robotic wheelchair; and γ is the side inclination and is related to angular velocity. Figure 2.2 shows the two angles, and the α angle and the γ angle are computed using the following equations:

$$\alpha = \cos^{-1} \frac{Gy}{G} \qquad\qquad (2.1)$$

$$\gamma = \cos^{-1} \frac{Gz}{G} \qquad\qquad (2.2)$$

2.3.2 Angle sensor

There are number of applications such as HCI and posture control devices that require measuring the angle of one or more joints. Goniometers are sensors that measure the angle of a joint and are based on the variable resistance potentiometer. A typical potentiometer has two ends, with one end connected to the base resistance and the other end is connected to the wiper that presses on the

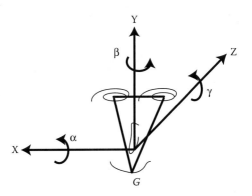

FIGURE 2.2   Computing head inclination angles.

base resistance, and the two ends determine the resistance between the two ends. The goniometer has two arms, with each of these connected with the two ends of the potentiometer, and the angle between these alters the resistance of the sensor. Generally, the relationship between the resistance and the angle is maintained to be nearly linear so that collaboration is relatively simple [13].

Goniometers have been in use for over five decades, and goniometers have been made smaller, lighter, and more robust. They have found number of applications such as for the control of braces and posture support devices. However, goniometers are being replaced by flexible angle sensors.

Sensors such as flex sensors are suitable for measuring angles of flexion (Figure 2.3) and angles of the neck. Flex sensors are inexpensive, easy to be used, and do not require any special setup. However, there does not appear to be a ready to be used system, and thus there is the need for building a small circuit and suitable software that will allow the use of such sensors for controlling a device such as the computer cursor or a wheelchair.

The flex sensor marketed by Spectra Symbol USA [13] changes the resistance when it is bent. When straight and not flexed, its nominal impedance is 10 kΩ, and increases to about 40 kΩ when bent in the middle at 90°, or right angle. The sensor is very flexible, and can be twisted and flexed greater than 360° as well.

Commonly available flex sensors are made of metal-coated polymer, with a length of 10.1 cm, width of 0.635 cm, and thickness of 0.05 cm. It has a single connector on one end, and its impedance is proportional to its angle. It is a very cost-effective, long-lasting, and easy to use device. In most such sensors, the change in the impedance is very significant and can be measured using the voltage divider network. Although the frequency of operation of these devices is relatively low in most applications, this is not important because rate of human movement is generally not greater than 1.5 Hz, which is achieved by elite cyclists.

Flexible angle sensors can be built into the garment of the user, such as a glove, socks, or knee bandage, and be used to determine the joint angles such as that of the elbow or identify finger flexion. Flexible angle sensors may also be integrated with other modalities such as the electromyogram. Information from both of these are fed into the computer or logic circuit to determine the direction and angle of the joint movement.

2.3.3 Stretch sensor   Development of conductive polymers has resulted in the development of stretch sensors, the resistance of which is proportional to its length. Typically, these sensors are polymers that have carbon infusion, and when these are stretched, the length increases while the diameter reduces. This results in an increase in the resistance, and measuring this change is an indicator of the length of the sensor [14–16].

One simple application of these sensors for people who lack hand control is to appropriately embed these sensors into a garment of the person such that the intended movement of the user causes stretch of the sensor. When suitably embedded in the headgear of the user, stretch sensors can identify the head movement toward the right, left or backward, and be used for controlling a computerized device.

The advantage of such sensors is that they are simple to use and are inexpensive. They also allow the user to personalize the device such that it can be used for people of different sizes, age groups, and allow them their own style of operation. However, there are no complete systems that are available, and the user or their caregiver has to custom build the system. This also makes such a system difficult for wireless operations.

2.3.4 Force sensor

There are a large number of force sensors, and these range from simple to very accurate. The cost and complexity of force sensors can vary significantly as well. One of the common issues with people having reduced motor control is that there force is not stable and well-controlled, and hence for most such applications, the high accuracy force sensors are not required [17,18].

One example of a force sensor is the Flexiforce [17]. It is a single-element force sensor and its electrical resistance changes with the applied force. When there is no force, and the force sensor is unloaded, its resistance is very high. When force is applied to the sensor, this resistance decreases. The sensor is provided with two electrical pins and the resistance between these pins can be measured using a simple electronic circuit. The relationship between the force and resistance is linear though this linearity is not accurate.

This sensor does not have the stability or accuracy for fine subtle gradation-based control and cannot distinguish between pressing forward on the stick a little bit and pushing it as far as it will go. However, it is suitable for identifying if the force is there or not, and thus its output is suitable for being binary. This is often very useful for people with limited control and thus can be incorporated in devices such as wheelchair control using head pressure. Such sensors are useful because they are flexible, lightweight, and inexpensive.

2.3.4.1 Example of smart glove The biomedical laboratory of RMIT University, Melbourne, Australia developed a smart glove (Figure 2.3) that can be used by people with weak muscles, or for performing tasks that may have the risk of injury. In the basic design, the smart glove has a network of sensors that identify hand and finger movement, which is used to control the robotic prosthetic hand.

The basic design consists of a glove that has sensors to identify the movement of each finger, the palm, and the wrist. For this purpose, 10 flex sensors (described earlier) were incorporated. These sensors measure the bending at the joint and were used for the following:

- Five sensors to identify finger flexion
- One sensor to identify thumb abduction/adduction
- One sensor to identify palm flexion
- One sensor for wrist flexion
- One sensor for wrist extension
- One sensor for radial and ulnar deviation

The required electronic circuit was built into the glove. The output of each sensor was multiplexed and digitized using low-resolution 4 bits and transmitted to the computer using a USB connection.

2.3.4.2 Computer connectivity specifics Sensors have to be connected to the computer and this is either done using a wired or wireless connection. The wireless connections have

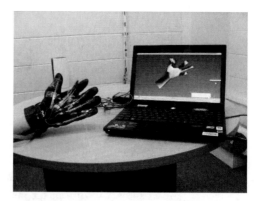

FIGURE 2.3 Smart glove for controlling the virtual hand developed at Biosignals Lab, RMIT University, Melbourne, Australia.

the obvious advantage that there are no wires, and this allows freedom to the user. Wireless also avoids the clutter of wires and this makes it easier to make changes to the configuration, which can be achieved by software. The wireless options may use Bluetooth or a wireless network approach. In each of these cases, each sensor can be individually addressed so that the system can read the sensors separately. However, wireless transmission consumes significant power, and when there are no wires, this requires the sensors to carry batteries, which makes them bulky.

Wired connections eliminate the need for battery power and the devices can draw on the power from the computer. As most mechanical sensor-based HCIs are low-frequency devices, a USB port is an efficient solution. This connection can be achieved using an electronic chip such as the Microchip PIC18F4550 to control the interface to the computer. This has a possible 32 inputs or 16 bidirectional inputs, and can be used for a significantly complex smart glove or similar device.

2.4 Applications of HCI based on mechanical sensors

HCI devices that are based on mechanical sensors have a number of advantages including simplicity and acceptability by the user. Such devices have been in common usage ever since graphics-based computing began and have been extensively developed, with most people very confident with their usage. Thus, the typical user does not require any extensive training and they can use these without delay.

Another significant advantage of these interfaces is that they are relatively inexpensive and available in all parts of the world. Further, most of these are compatible with existing drivers or computer software, and are often referred to as plug-and-play type. Thus, the user can plug the device to their computer or other such equipment and use it with no extra effort.

Mechanical sensor-based HCI have the advantage that many technical people are comfortable in customizing and servicing such equipment. Thus, if the specific device is not directly suitable for the user, technical support personnel can customize it. They also have the advantage of being robust and reliable, and are generally immune to factors such as electromagnetic interference. Thus, such devices are the most commonly used computer interface devices.

2.4.1 Shortcomings of HCI based on mechanical sensors

Mechanical sensing is based on movement or force and thus necessitates the user to make some movement or exert force. This limits the use of these devices for those users who have some level of muscle control and contraction. Hence, mechanical sensor-based HCI are unsuitable for people who do not have hand or leg movement or control, such as spinal cord injured patients who may have lack of motor control. Thus, this is not useful for people who may be quadriplegic.

2.5 Current research and future improvements

There has been significant advancement in material engineering over the recent past. Current techniques can develop materials with specific thermal, electrical, and mechanical properties. Thus, devices such as joysticks or tracking balls can be built with specific weights, friction, and electrical properties, and conductive polymers with elastic or bend properties have led to the ability to sense position, stretch, and angle [19].

Another recent advancement in the field of mechanical development is the 3D printer. With easy availability of these printers, it is relatively simple to produce customized objects and parts that can be used to customize computer interface devices such as a joystick. Although this would have required significant engineering effort earlier, the printer can produce most objects based on the computer-based design [20].

Efforts have also been made for the mechanical sensors to be fabricated using biocompatible materials. This, coupled with wireless technology that allows power and data transmission, has found applications in implanted sensors required to monitor orthopedic implants such as for bones and joints. Such sensors will reduce the need for unnecessary surgical procedures and enhance the life of the implants, thereby greatly improving the quality of life of the users.

References

1. KARRAY F, ALEMZADEH M, ABOUSALEH J, NOURS ARAB M. Human–computer interaction: Overview on state of the art. *International Journal on Smart Sensing and Intelligent Systems* 2008:1(1), 137–159.
2. SHIH C-H, SHIH C-T. Assisting people with multiple disabilities to use computers with multiple mice. *Research in Developmental Disabilities* 2009:30(4), 746–754.

3. KARLQVIST L, BERNMARK E, EKENVALL L, HAGBERG M, ISAKSSON A, ROSTÖ T. Computer mouse and track-ball operation: Similarities and differences in posture, muscular load and perceived exertion. *International Journal of Industrial Ergonomics* 1999:23(3), 157–169.

4. SONG Y, ZHANG Y, WANG Z, XIE P. The head-trace mouse for elderly: A human–computer interaction system based on detection of poses of head and mouth. *International Journal of Information Technology* 2013:19(2), 1–13.

5. YANCO HA. Wheelesley: A robotic wheelchair system: Indoor navigation and user interface. *Assistive Technology and AI, LNAI* 1998:1458, 256–268.

6. BUXTON W, HILL R, ROWLEY P. Issues and techniques in touch-sensitive tablet input. *Computer Graphics* 1985:19(3), 215–223.

7. PEREIRA CAM, NETO RB, REYNALDO AC, DE MIRANDA LUZO MC, OLIVEIRA RP. Development and evaluation of a head-controlled human–computer interface with mouse-like functions for physically disabled users. *Clinics (Sao Paulo, Brazil)* 2009:64(10), 975–981.

8. JACK D, BOIAN R, MERIANS AS, TREMAINE M, BURDEA GC, ADAMOVICH SV, RECCE M, POIZNER H. Virtual reality-enhanced stroke rehabilitation. *IEEE Transactions on Neural Systems and Rehabilitation Engineering* 2001:9(3), 308–318.

9. COOPER RA. Intelligent control of power wheelchairs. *IEEE Engineering in Medicine and Biology Magazine* 1995: 14(4), 423–431.

10. KUMAR P, RAUTARAY SS, AGRAWAL A. Hand data glove: A new generation real-time mouse for Human-Computer Interaction. 1st International Conference on Recent Advances in Information Technology (RAIT) 2012: 750–755.

11. BENBASAT AY, PARADISO JA. An inertial measurement framework for gesture recognition and applications, gesture and sign language in human–computer interaction. *Lecture Notes in Computer Science* 2002:2298, 9–20.

12. BASTOS-FILHO T, FERREIRA A, CAVALIERI D, SILVA R, MULLER S, PEREZ E. Multi-modal interface for communication operated by eye blinks, eye movements, head movements, blowing/sucking and brain waves. *IEEE ISSNIP Biosignals and Biorobotics Conference* (BRC) 2013: 1–6.

13. MORITANI H, KAWAI Y, SAWADA H. Intuitive manipulation of a haptic monitor for the gestural human–computer interaction, gesture-based communication in human-computer interaction. *Lecture Notes in Computer Science* 2004:2915, 386–398.

14. Flex Sensor. Spectra Symbol USA. Available at: http://www.spectrasymbol.com/wp-Content/themes/spectra/images/datasheets/FlexSensor.pdf. Accessed December 9, 2014.

15. FARRINGDON J, MOORE AJ, TILBURY N, CHURCH J, BIEMOND PD. Wearable sensor badge and sensor jacket for context awareness. *The Third International Symposium on Wearable Computers* 1999: 107–113.

16. StretchSense Limited. New Zealand. Available at: http://www.stretchsense.com/. Accessed December 9, 2014.

17. O'BRIEN B, GISBY T, ANDERSON, IA. Stretch sensors for human body motion. *Proceedings of SPIE 9056, Electroactive Polymer Actuators and Devices (EAPAD)* 2014: 1–9.

18. Tekscan. Force Sensors. Available at: http://www.tekscan.com/flexible-force-sensors. Accessed December 9, 2014.

19. MORGANTI E, ANGELINI L, ADAMI A, LALANNE D, LORENZELLI L, MUGELLINI E. A smart watch with embedded sensors to recognize objects, grasps and forearm gestures. *Procedia Engine*ering 2012:41,1169–1175.

20. RAUTARAY SS, AGRAWAL A. Vision based hand gesture recognition for human computer interaction: A survey. *Artificial Intelligence Review* 2012:43(1), 1–54.

CHAPTER THREE

Brain–computer interface based on thought waves

Abstract

Our actions are thought in the brain, and the movement is implemented by the combination of neural transmission and muscle activation. Similarly, our sensing is perceived by us by our brain receiving the neural signals from our sensory organs. However, many people do not have functioning neural pathways or muscles that produce sufficient force. For such people, technology that connects the muscles or sensory organs directly with the brain is referred to as brain–computer interface (BCI). Such connectivity may be achieved using invasive or noninvasive methods.

This chapter describes the use of brain waves recorded by noninvasive and invasive techniques to produce an action command. In this chapter, the fundamentals of brain waves, the electroencephalogram or electroencephalography (EEG), and BCI are introduced. Subsequently, EEG recording and analysis technology is described and the methods for automatic identification of commands from EEG are discussed. This chapter also briefly explains sensory BCI devices.

Current technologies and implementation are then described along with the possible applications, user requirements, and limitations. In the end of this chapter, some of the major current and proposed research activities are discussed.

3.1 Introduction

Our actions are controlled by the brain, and the process of people controlling devices can be described in terms of our thoughts being converted to neural activity in the brain, and these cause activation of the muscles, which leads to movement. This is translated by the interface such as the joystick or computer mouse to the command of the machine. The feedback of the movement is obtained by the user and this is used to control the action and make corrections. Thus, controlling a machine or a computer requires a healthy spinal and peripheral neural system and muscles, as well as a healthy sensory system. However, people who may have suffered injuries to their spine or suffer muscular atrophy are unable to perform such actions. Similar communication is difficult, and people with such ailments may be unable to speak or write, and thus are locked in their bodies unable to communicate with the rest of the world. BCI systems have been developed to provide the direct interface between the brain of an individual with a computer or a peripheral device. The other aim is to provide the users with the ability to sense when they have lost some of their sensory capabilities.

A BCI is a communication system that does not depend on peripheral nerves and muscles [1]. BCI describes a set of devices or technologies that allow the user to control and command a computer with only brain waves. It is also a term that is used for technologies that allow the user to obtain sensory information directly to their brain without the sensory nerves or senses. These are the outcomes of decades of intensive research that has improved the understanding of the functioning of the brain, along with advances in signal processing, electronics, and computers. BCI provides the user the capacity to interface with the computer for commanding or receiving information. Thus, BCI provides users the ability to hear, touch, and see when they have lost their natural abilities to perform these functions, and to give commands to machines directly from the brain, and thus give the user the capacity to convert their thought to actions.

BCI devices may be broadly divided into two categories: feedback or sensory, and feedforward or motor. Motor BCI enables a direct communications pathway between the brain and the object to be controlled. The signal is directly transmitted from the brain to the mechanism directing the cursor, rather than taking the normal route through the body's neuromuscular system from the brain to the finger on a mouse.

There are number of motor BCI techniques and can be divided into two categories: thought-based passive and simulated systems. Thought-based systems are often referred to as thought translation devices (TTDs), and is the focus of this chapter.

The BCI may be achieved using invasive or noninvasive techniques. The invasive systems have the advantage that the electrodes are placed directly on the brain, and the signal recording is more precise. However, these systems require extensive surgery and more complex equipment due to issues such as biocompatibility, reliability, and power. There is also invasive BCI where the electrodes are implanted without major brain surgery and these are now regularly being used for giving sensory information to the user. The cochlear implant is an example of a success story. Devices for commanding a computer or other devices are still in the very early stages, and being trialed on primates or extreme cases. Noninvasive systems, however, are relatively inexpensive and are easy to install on the user but lack precision.

By reading signals from an array of neurons and using computer chips and programs to translate the signals into action, BCI can enable a person suffering from paralysis to write a book or control a motorized wheelchair or prosthetic limb through thought alone. Current brain–interface devices require deliberate conscious thought; some future applications, such as prosthetic control, are likely to work effortlessly. One of the biggest challenges in developing BCI technology has been the development of electrode devices and surgical methods that are minimally invasive. In the traditional BCI model, the brain accepts an implanted mechanical device and controls the device as a natural part of its representation of the body. Much of the current research is focused on the potential on noninvasive BCI.

3.2 History of brain–computer interface

An EEG is the recording of the electrical activity of the brain. This was first observed by Hans Berger in 1924 and has since found numerous applications, including the development of BCI. The early applications of EEG were largely clinical, such as for epilepsy, but soon were followed by other applications such as modeling the brain and for discovering the relationship between human motor and sensory perception with the electrical activity of the brain. In the 1960s, it was observed that

EEG recorded from the scalp could be associated with thought, stress, and concentration patterns, and in 1970 came the first attempt for the development of thought-driven BCI. Since then, researchers have reported the motor mapping, where the location of the brain was mapped to various motor and sensory functions. Algorithms were developed that could identify the motor thoughts directly from EEG recordings.

In the 1970s, several scientists developed simple communication systems that were driven by electrical activity recorded from the head. Early in 1970s, the U.S. Department of Defense, through its research arm Advanced Research Projects Agency (ARPA), supported research in these technologies with the intent to develop technologies that provided an immersive and intimate interaction between human and machines or computers, referred to as "bionic" applications.

One of the pioneers in this bionic research was the work by Dr. George Lawrence [2], which focused on cognitive biofeedback and self-regulation. This project worked toward biofeedback techniques to enhance the human performance and capability, especially for military personnel. The specific project aim was to support tasks that caused mental fatigue and had high mental loads. The research resulted in improved understanding of human motor control system, specifically in sensory feedback and biofeedback. Although this was pioneering work, the outcomes were only preliminary.

Another important pioneering project in this area was "Biocybernetics." This was established to evaluate the use of bioelectrical signals such as EEG to control devices for defense and other applications, especially to assist in the control of vehicles and weapons, or other similar systems. The Brain–Computer Interface Laboratory at the University of California in Los Angles (UCLA) demonstrated the use of visual evoked potentials (VEPs) [3,4] to identify the direction of the gaze of the user, and thus provide the human with the ability to control the movement of a cursor. An important outcome of these studies was that they were able to distinguish between EEG and muscle activity of the scalp, and highlighted the difference and similarity between EEG activity and those using electromyogram (EMG) recorded from the scalp.

Implanting electrodes in the brain was first attempted in 1960s when the electrical activity of the brain was recorded directly from the brain surface. These works identified the location of the motor cortex and auditory centers, and correlated the actions and sensory stimulation with the help of animal experiments. Experiments were conducted to stimulate the sensory regions of the brain for perception of sensory functions, such as sound. The auditory center was extensively studied and led to the development of cochlear implants.

Extensive research with the help of animal experiments was performed in 1970s, and building on earlier work, brain stimulation for sensory perception and motor mapping was demonstrated [5,6]. These works demonstrated the advantages of embedded systems compared with the surface recordings of EEG, and showed that these recordings were more precise and repeatable, while the precision was lacking in EEG recorded from the scalp of the person. However, there were significant limitations such as the size of the electronics, wires, and surgical procedures that limited progress in the development of BCI devices that could be directly placed on the cortex.

After the 1960s, several mysteries of the brain was uncovered such as the functioning of the motor cortex, which resulted in developing procedures for placements of electrodes and association of the limb with electrode location. These were the basis for the first series of significant intracortical BCI that were developed in the 1990s. In early 2000, the first experiments were conducted where the lab monkeys' movements were reproduced by the robotic arm with only the connectivity to the cortex [7,8].

There have also been significant research and development focused on neuroprosthetic applications that aim at restoring damaged hearing, sight, and movement. Due to the remarkable cortical plasticity of the brain, signals from implanted prostheses, after adaptation, can be handled by the brain like natural sensor or effector channels. Following years of animal experimentation, the first neuroprosthetic devices implanted in humans appeared in the mid-1990s.

The first human experiment was conducted at Emory University in Atlanta, which was the first to report the recording of signals from electrodes implanted in the brain and to simulate movement in 1998. The patient, however, did not live long, but just long enough to start working with the implant, eventually learning to control a computer cursor [9].

There has been significant progress in noninvasive, scalp EEG-based BCI. Until around 2000, these devices were largely limited to the laboratory due to the prohibitive cost of EEG recording devices, wires, and size of the electronics, but there has been significant improvement since then. Devices such as the EPOC headset by Emotiv Company were introduced, and are inexpensive as well as easy to wear, and became popular with computer gamers, and found applications for people with disabilities. Faster and smaller computer devices have also contributed to making these devices available outside the laboratory. The availability of tablets and laptops that are easy to mount on wheelchairs and with sufficient computation power have made it possible for these devices to be deployed.

3.3 Significance of BCI devices

There are two major types of BCI machines: sensory and motor. Thanks to the success of the cochlear implant, the sensory BCI does not require much introduction. The technology has come a long way from the start and now over millions of people have a cochlear implant. However, it is worth noting that the implant was the brainchild of an Australian scientist Graeme Clark, who in Melbourne developed the first implant device that was fitted for Rod Saunders in 1978. This was truly sensational and has been responsible for changing the perception of bionic devices in the minds of laymen and scientists. However, it should be noted that this was the outcome of global efforts and many changes to the direction of the technology.

Motor BCI machines have had smaller success, and while success has been reported and papers published during the past 50 years, demonstrated success has only been more recent. Some of the recent high-profile users of BCI have brought public and political attention to these devices. One such example was in 2006 when at the European Research and Innovation Exhibition in Paris, Dr. Brunner (from the United States) composed a message on the screen by thinking his thoughts alone. He wore a noninvasive cap with electrodes placed on his scalp and EEG activity was recorded and analyzed. The software with a range of algorithms identified the specific characters to type the message [10].

BCI systems like that demonstrated by Brunner use a set of algorithms and pattern-matching techniques to identify the user commands. The systems have to be adaptive to ensure the signal quality, has to be customized to the individual, and the user is able to become more efficient with practice. The effectiveness of the technology is evidenced by the ability of the user to communicate effectively and thus be an integral member of the society. Although the user is unable to make any movement, including eye movement, this provides the user with the ability to communicate effectively and thus not suffer locked-in syndrome. The following example highlights this point.

An American neurobiologist despite having suffered from amyotrophic lateral sclerosis (Lou Gehrig's disease) and not able to move his eyes, was able to e-mail: "I am a neuroscientist who (sic) couldn't work without BCI. I am writing this with my EEG courtesy of the Wadsworth Center Brain-Computer Interface Research Program." [10].

Another successful application of TTD-based BCI devices is their use for applications for controlling devices such as wheelchairs. There are several research teams, including at the University Espirito Santo, Vitoria, and Brazil, that have successfully integrated the TTD to control wheelchairs and have tested these for quadriplegic patients. Restoring the ability of an individual to maneuver a wheelchair and gain independence highlights the outcome of this technology.

3.4 BCI technology

BCI is an output channel for the brain, which is new to the user, who has to be trained for using the system. It requires the user to engage the brain's adaptive capacities and adjust output to optimize performance. Its operation depends on the interaction of two adaptive and seemingly independent controllers: the user's brain, which produces the brain waves, and the system itself, which translates the activity into specific commands. Successful BCI operation requires the user to develop a new skill to control the EEG without the feedback of associated muscle activity.

BCI can be broadly considered into two categories: invasive and noninvasive. Invasive BCI have electrodes that are implanted in the brain of the user, and noninvasive BCI have electrodes that are on the surface. These are described next.

3.4.1 Invasive BCI
Invasive BCIs are implanted directly into the brain during neurosurgery, and are able to obtain the signal directly from the neurons or directly stimulate the neurons. The biggest advantage of implanted devices is high specificity as these devices are in direct contact with the neurons. These devices can be classified into motor and sensory.

3.4.2 Motor-invasive BCI
For BCI that are for the purpose of obtaining the motor commands from the user, the motor cortex is the obvious choice for placing the electrodes. This is because its relevance to the motor tasks, and also relative accessibility being located on the brain surface, compared to deeper located motor areas in the brain. It is

also more convenient due to the large pyramidal cells. Alternate sites such as the supplementary motor cortex, subcortical motor areas, and the thalamus have also been considered.

Numerous modalities have been considered for stimulating the brain including functional magnetic resonance imaging (fMRI) and magnetoencephalography (MEG), besides the electrical stimulation. There are also the use of electrocorticography (ECoG), which is less invasive, and in this modality, the electrical activity of the brain is recorded from beneath the skull but in a manner similar to noninvasive electroencephalography. The electrodes are embedded in a thin (biocompatible flexible polymer) pad that is placed above the cortex and under the dura mater.

The suitable locations of the electrodes are obtained using imaging techniques such as fMRI and high-density EEG electrodes [11,12]. However, there are numerous unknowns in these systems, such as how many neurons are required to obtain the recordings, the possible role of stimulation of the region to modify the region response, and the ability of the user to retrain the brain based on the known plasticity in the neural connections. There are conflicting views regarding each of these, and significant research is required to reach the best answer.

There are also ethical issues associated with invasive BCI. This involves highly invasive procedures that would significantly alter natural brain functioning, and thus to be justifiable, an implanted system must offer the individual a substantial functional advantage over conventional augmentative technologies and over noninvasive BCI methods. If, for example, improved noninvasive techniques can provide a simple hand grasp compared with precise grips with an invasive procedure, are such options justified? Often, there are no simple answers. However, amyotrophic lateral sclerosis (ALS) patients who are locked in, and selected patients suffering from stroke or spinal cord injury, may benefit from invasive BCI technology if it is both safe and effective.

For effective motor BCI operation, the system must also provide sensory information to the user when the body's natural ability to obtain this information is defective. The nervous system's ability to adapt to the new feedback provided by a BCI helps the user to effectively command the devices. There are also many other applications of the sensory BCI, such as the auditory, and more recently the visual prostheses.

3.4.3 Noninvasive BCI

Noninvasive BCI is largely for motor command function detection, and there are no significant works in its application for sensory applications. Such BCI is also referred to as TTD. The noninvasive nature and user convenience are its strengths, though the lack of specificity is the biggest weakness. The fundamental principle of these devices is based on the electrical or magnetic recording corresponding to the brain activity of the user.

EEG is the recording of the electrical activity of the brain, recorded from the scalp of the person. In conventional scalp EEG, the recording is obtained by placing electrodes on the scalp with a conductive gel. Many systems typically use electrodes, each of which is attached to an individual wire, though more recently, wireless electrodes are becoming common. EEG was discovered in 1924 and has extensively been used for a number of clinical applications such as epilepsy [13]. It has also been a very important tool in our understanding of brain functioning.

EEG is a low voltage, low frequency signal, with signal amplitude being around 1 microvolt, and the frequency being in the range of 0–100 Hz, though the effective frequency is in the range of 0.5–50 Hz. While traditional EEG uses 19 electrodes with 1 reference electrode, there are many other options that have been recently developed. One of the options is the use of high-density electrodes, where as many as 256 electrodes are placed on the scalp to obtain greater detail and specificity of the signal [12].

Traditionally, EEG analysis was done based on the spectral content, with the signal being divided into five frequency bands: alpha, beta1, beta2, gamma, and theta. However, with advancement in electronics and signal processing techniques, there are many other options that are now available. The other method of obtaining the information regarding the brain activity is the use of MEG. MEG detects the tiny magnetic fields created as neurons within the brain. It has been found to identify the location of the active region and can be used for determining the command of the user. However, this appears to be confined to laboratory research.

3.5 System design

BCI systems have evolved over the years, largely due to the miniaturization of the electronics, improved computation devices, advancements in algorithms, and improved surgical procedures. The system design for the invasive and noninvasive devices is significantly different, and so is the difference between the sensory and motor devices. The basic system requirements are discussed in the next sections.

3.5.1 Invasive thought translation device BCI

Such a device requires the implanted electrodes that record the activity from the appropriate locations. These devices have to be connected with the external recording system, and due to the obvious issue of infections, wired connections are difficult. Thus, the desired option is for these electrodes to be connected wirelessly. However, the thickness of the skull, and presence of blood with hemoglobin makes the wireless connectivity challenging.

The other key component of invasive TTD is the signal analysis and classification system, and the ability to train the system for the individual user. With the easy availability of miniaturized computers, this is no longer a significant challenge.

3.5.2 Invasive sensory BCI

Sensory BCI requires a combination of the sensory device, such as the microphone, the signal analysis and classification system, and the electrodes that are implanted appropriately in the brain. In some text, devices such as cochlear are not referred to as BCI because the electrode placement may not be considered as part of the brain. With this industry having matured, this procedure is now well rehearsed and no longer considered highly invasive. In this system, there are around 24 electrodes, located on a single wire that is introduced in the cochlear and stimulated externally based on the microphone.

3.5.3 Noninvasive thought translation device BCI

Noninvasive TTDs are typically based on the recording of EEG from the scalp. While earlier devices required the use of EEG cap, some of the new devices uses head-sets that are easy to place, and do not have the appearance of a clinical product.

Advancements in signal processing and motor mapping have resulted in reducing the number of channels that are required for obtaining the necessary information. Some of the current devices are based only on eight electrodes, though the earlier devices used significantly more number of channels. Current devices have also evolved to have the electrodes that are wireless and that are able to self-monitor the connectivity between the electrode and the skin surface.

One key component for the devices is the computer and the software that can be trained for the specific user. The current technologies often require significant manual supervision by an expert to train the system such that the system can correctly interpret the user command. Often, techniques such as neural networks or statistical classifiers are used for this purpose.

One key component of all TTD BCI devices is the robotic or communication device that will be controlled by the user. With limitations such as the degrees of freedom for the user, it is essential that the devices such as the keyboard (screen) have to be simplified. There is also the limitation regarding the language skills. Some of the systems to overcome the short-comings include the use of icon-based keyboards that allow the keyboard to be tailored to the user requirements, are not language based, and require fewer degrees of freedom compared with a normal keyboard.

3.6 Signal analysis

Interpreting the brain waves to determine the user's thought is the aim of the signal analysis and classification. One of the first challenges is to reduce the noise and obtain the signal that is suitable for analysis. Thus, the first goal of signal analysis is to maximize the signal-to-noise ratio (SNR) of the EEG. This requires an understanding of the major sources of noise. After the signal quality has been improved, the next task is to identify and obtain the most suitable set of signal features that can be interpreted to determine the user thought command.

3.6.1 Improving signal quality

There are number of sources of noise such as due to eye movements, EMG, and line noise (50 Hz). There are also other sources of EEG that are not relevant to the application and may be inherent or due to distractions. Discriminating to identify the relevant signal and the noise is always the biggest challenge when the characteristics of the noise are similar in frequency, time, or amplitude to those of the desired signal. For example, eye movements are of greater concern than EMG when a slow cortical potential is the BCI input feature because eye movements and slow potentials have overlapping frequency ranges. For the same reason, EMG is of greater concern than eye movements when a rhythm is the input feature. In the laboratory, particularly, it is important to record enough information (e.g., topographical and spectral distributions) to permit discrimination between signal and noise.

Nonneural noise such as EMG is of particular concern because a user's control over it can readily masquerade as actual EEG control. Nonneural noise produced by reflex activity may occur even in users who lack all voluntary muscle control. In this case, the nonneural noise will not support communication but can degrade BCI performance by reducing the SNR. It is also important to distinguish between different neural features. The visual rhythm is a source of noise when the rhythm is the feature being used for communication.

Temporal and spectral filtering are two important methods used for signal analysis. However, spectral and temporal overlap of multiple signals and signal with noise is inherent in EEG recordings and this limits the outcome. More recently, approaches such as independent component analysis and other entropy and information-based techniques have been employed to separate the signal from background noise and noise due to other sources.

3.6.2 EEG feature selection

There are many options for features of BCI signal processing, and the efficacy of each is application based. These have to be evaluated based on speed, accuracy, and ease for the user training. There are online tools that have been built such as BCI-Matlab [14] and Graz BCI system [15]. One method that has been successfully employed is autoregressive (AR) model parameter estimation, useful for describing EEG activity and BCI applications. It typically assumes a Gaussian process [16], and it is important to assess the signal for this technique to be successful. An alternate is the maximum likelihood estimate or Kalman filter approach [17].

Signal processing and classification methods are very critical in BCI design. After enhancing the SNR, the suitable features of the signal have to be obtained. However, the human brain is complex, and undergoes other changes such as motivation, intention, frustration, fatigue, and learning, and these significantly affect the signal.

3.7 BCI translation algorithms

A translation algorithm transforms the EEG features into device control commands. These classify the signal feature set based on prior knowledge of the relationship between the user commands and the signal features. There are several options for classifying signals such as EEG, and these are based on factors such as the speed of training, speed of classification, sensitivity, specificity, accuracy, number of samples, and statistical distribution of the data. Because some of the factors are counterinteractions, a compromise between them is required, and for this purpose, a thorough understanding of the application is essential. For example, if the device is required for a single user, the speed of training may not be a critical factor because retraining of the system is not required. Moreover, if the system does not provide the user with feedback, it is essential for the system specificity to be very high.

Translation algorithms that have been used including linear discriminate analysis (LDA), neural networks, Bayesian classifiers, support vector machine (SVM), and twin support vector machine (T-SVM). These have their individual strengths and weakness and need to be carefully evaluated for best performance for an application.

3.8 User consideration

BCI devices are not suitable for all people. TTDs can be limited to who can use the device and the external conditions. Hair can lead to reduced conductivity and the recording may be corrupted due to the presence of line noise and motion artifacts. There is also the concern about the language, emotions, and inability of some users to get trained to repeatedly generate the appropriate EEG. There are also concerns regarding the ability of the user to understand the request from the clinician when they are training the system, while others may have difficulty due to added impairments such as hearing or visual loss.

Matching the user with his or her optimal BCI input features is essential if BCIs are ever to be broadly applied to the communication needs of users with different disabilities. There are inherent weakness of the BCI systems, and in some cases, a hybrid approach may be more suitable.

3.9 Applications of BCI

BCI provides the user the ability to interact with a computerized machine without requiring any movement or even activation of the muscles or motor nerves. Such a system will be useful for disabled people, people in special situations such as defense, computer games, and entertainment. The highest impact will be for facilitating communication for people with disabilities such as quadriplegics. These people often find themselves totally locked in with no means to communicate with the outside world, and this can be extremely frustrating.

Although BCI is a generic name for a set of devices that allow the user to control computers or communicate directly from the brain and without muscle control, this chapter specifically refers to devices that are controlled by the thoughts of the user and are referred to as TTD. TTDs can be invasive and noninvasive. Each of these is described in the next sections.

3.9.1 Applications of invasive TTD The invasive sensory devices have progressed significantly more than TTDs. One of the biggest successes is the cochlear device, which is now routinely used for people who have impaired hearing. Its success has resulted in optimism and research groups around the world are working toward the bionic eye, where it is envisaged that the retina will be replaced by a silicon device.

Invasive TTDs are still in the very early stages, and thus most experiments have been conducted only on animals. However, more recently, they have been implanted in people who are referred to as totally locked-in, such as ALS patients, who progressively lose all motor control functions. Totally locked-in patients are those who do not have any voluntary muscle functions, and are unable to perform tasks such as speech, eye or eyelid movement, or control air-suck and push functions. Certain acquired brain injury and spinal cord injury patients may also be in a similar category. Because of the extreme nature of their situation, such invasive procedures have been attempted for their benefits. From the results, it is evident that it is important for the implants to be provided prior to these patients losing all or most of their voluntary functions, because subsequently it is difficult training these patients to learn to use the device.

Future applications of invasive TTDs are expected to be for a range of disorders including autism, aphasia, and other severe communication disorders. This is because TTD allows the bypass of the region of the brain that may have been compromised.

3.9.2 Applications of noninvasive TTD Noninvasive TTDs are based on the use of EEG. The applications of these are more widespread. The advantage of such a system is that it is relatively easy to install and does not require any surgical procedure. There are devices such as EPOC (Emotiv) that are easy to wear, look attractive, are simple to calibrate, and cost under $1000. These properties make these easy to afford and user friendly. Although these devices provide the user with very few degrees of freedom, the aforementioned advantages make them highly accessible and are being widely used. The early stage applications of these have largely been for entertainment and computer games, and have paved the way for communication devices for people who have highly impaired motor control, such as road trauma patients who may have suffered spinal cord injuries.

Noninvasive TTD

- Allows those with disabilities to communicate, control devices such as a light switch and wheelchair, and the ability to play computer games.
- Provides enhanced channels for healthy users when controlling computer games or similar devices.
- Controls robotic devices for health or entertainment applications.
- Provides feedback to users with sensory loss.

Future applications of these devices include the use of BCI for defense applications such as guiding weapons or controlling a vehicle.

3.10 Limitations

Invasive TTDs have several limitations, the biggest being the highly noninvasive nature of the procedure. Although researchers have been working on simplifying the procedure and reducing the uncertainty, there are significant unknowns prior to the procedure, making it difficult to predict the outcomes. Another unknown is the long-term effect of the devices in the brain, due to growth of tissues around the electrodes.

Another limitation is the inability of some of the users to use the device. Results demonstrate that it is important for the patients to begin using these devices before they lose their voluntary functions. This is a serious limitation, because prior to the complete loss, implanting such devices is ethically challenging. The other limitation is that such patients lose their ability to sense, and thus appropriate feedback has to be given to such patients. The users have to be trained to provide feedback to the user using a different set of modalities than would be natural, and the user may not be able to recognize this after the disease has progressed.

The noninvasive TTDs have limitations that are associated with very few degrees of freedom, poor reliability, and rapid changes to the signal quality over time. Although surface EEG-based TTDs have been shown to be suitable for controlling devices such as the wheelchair or the computer cursor on the screen, experimental results show that for most people, even four commands are difficult and anything more than that is not possible.

Although success of BCI systems is very evident, one of the biggest limitations is that they are relatively low bandwidth devices, offering maximum information transfer rates of 5–25 bits/min at best. Thus, the ability of the user to communicate is highly limited. To overcome this limitation, attempts have been made to change the keyboard that is displayed and provide the user with suitable icons. This has the limitation that it has to be customized for the individual user; however, it has the strength that the communication rate is greatly enhanced. It also overcomes the need for overcoming language boundaries.

One challenge to surface EEG systems is that the presence of hair causes significant changes to the electrode-skin impedance, resulting in altering the signal quality. Further, the presence of sweat or drying of the gel can lead to significant deterioration in the signal quality, and thus erroneous outcomes. The presence of hanging wires is another major shortcoming, though many research groups have partially solved this problem, and now wireless electrodes are expected to be soon available.

One common shortcoming in all TTDs is that the user has to make conscious thoughts to control the device while performing other activities. Thus, they have to manage their EEG, must simultaneously plan the message to be communicated, and select specific letters or cursor movements. They also have to observe the outcomes and initiate appropriate corrections where relevant. This requires the user to perform multitasking, and diversion of attention. These can limit the applications of such technologies.

3.11 Future research

The brain is considered the last challenge and the most complex part of the universe. Research groups have been working to better understand brain functioning and to develop techniques to interface directly with the brain. The list of projects is too long, but some of the interesting ones are as follows:

- Bionic eye—The bionic eye is a project that is supported by research organizations around the globe, and early stage progress has been reported. There are already experiments where the device has been implanted and results appear to be promising. However, there appears to be a number of challenges that would have to be overcome before we can hope that a blind person will have functional vision restored.

- Thought capture—To determine what the person is thinking. This may have many applications for defense, as well as for people with disabilities who would be able to communicate with the outside world. However, the progress of such projects appears to be highly limited.

- Dream capture—The aim of this project is to identify what the person is dreaming. This may be considered as an extension of thought capture, and the progress does not suggest that it will be available in the near future.

- There are also projects where organizations such as Google are attempting to perform large-scale data analysis of the brain map. However, details of this appear to be shrouded in secrecy.

3.12 Ethical consideration

There are a number of ethical issues that must be considered in implanting and recording electrodes in human volunteers. Patients must be informed of the risks and potential benefits of any intervention, especially an invasive procedure with uncertain benefit to the individual and possibly serious risks. Volunteers with severe disabilities may tend to greatly overestimate the potential benefits, so that risks and uncertainties must be clearly and forcefully explained. However, many people may want to volunteer for research that provides no direct benefit to them beyond the knowledge that they are participating in a research project that might help others with similar conditions in the future. They should not be denied this opportunity. The Belmont Report [18] enunciates three basic ethical standards for the conduct of human research.

- The first standard, respect for persons, incorporates the idea that individuals are autonomous agents and should be free to make their own choice regarding participation after being given a full understanding of the risks and benefits.

- The second standard, beneficence, obligates the investigator to act in a way that will maximize benefit to the individual volunteer and/or the greater society while simultaneously minimizing the risk of harm.

- The third standard, justice, obligates the investigator to design studies so that the benefits and burdens of research are shared in a just way. An ethicist should be involved in the earliest phases of any human research developing or testing invasive BCI methods.

References

1. WOLPAW JR, BIRBAUMER N, MCFARLAND DJ, PFURTSCHELLER G, VAUGHAN TM. Brain–computer interfaces for communication and control. *Clinical Neurophysiology* 2002:113(6), 767–791.
2. LAWRENCE GH. Biofeedback and performance: An update, final technical rept. Army Research Inst for the Behavioral and Social Sciences, 1984.
3. VIDAL JJ. Toward direct brain–computer communication. *Annual Review of Biophysics and Bioengineering* 1973:2(1), 157–180.
4. VIDAL JJ. Real-time detection of brain events in EEG. *Proceedings of the IEEE* 1977:65(5), 633.
5. TRAVERSA R, CICINELLI P, BASSI A, ROSSINI PM, BERNARDI GM. Mapping of motor cortical reorganization after stroke: A brain stimulation study with focal magnetic pulses. *Stroke* 1997:28, 110–117.
6. HANSON T, FITZSIMMONS N, O'DOHERTY JE. Technology for multielectrode micro stimulation of brain tissue. In *Methods for Neural Ensemble Recordings*, 2nd Edition, edited by Nicolelis MAL, 47–55. CRC Press, Boca Raton, FL, 2007.
7. WESSBERG J, STAMBAUGH CR, KRALIK JD, BECK PD, LAUBACH M et al. Real-time prediction of hand trajectory by ensembles of cortical neurons in primates. *Nature* 2008:408, 361–365.
8. CARMENA JM, LEBEDEV MA, CRIST RE, O'DOHERTY JE, SANTUCCI DM et al. Learning to control a brain–machine interface for reaching and grasping by primates. *PLoS Biology* 2003:1(2), e42.
9. KENNEDY PR, BAKAY RA. Restoration of neural output from a paralyzed patient by a direct brain connection. *Neuroreport* 1998:9(8), 1707–1711.
10. BRUNNER C, ANDREONI G, BIANCHI L, BLANKERTZ B, BREITWIESER C, KANOH S, KOTHE CA et al. BCI software platforms. In *Towards Practical Brain–Computer Interfaces*, edited by BZ Allison, S Dunne, R Leeb, JDR Millan, and A Nijholt, 303–331. Springer, Berlin, 2013.
11. SULZER J, HALLER S, SCHARNOWSKI F, WEISKOPF N, BIRBAUMER N, BLEFARI ML, BRUEHL AB et al. Real-time fMRI neurofeedback: Progress and challenges. *NeuroImage* 2013:76, 386–399.
12. CINCOTTI F, MATTIA D, ALOISE F, BUFALARI S, ASTOLFI L, DE VICOFALLANI F, TOCCI A et al. High-resolution EEG techniques for brain–computer interface applications. *Journal of Neuroscience Methods* 2008:167(1), 31–42.
13. BRONZINO JD. Principles of electroencephalography. In *The Biomedical Engineering Handbook*, edited by JD Bronzino, 201–212. CRC Press, Boca Raton, FL, 1995.

14. EDLINGER G. The brain-computer interface: Using MATLAB and Simulink for biosignal acquisition and processing. Mathworks Inc., 2006.

15. PFURTSCHELLER G, NEUPER C, MULLER GR, OBERMAIER B, KRAUSZ G, SCHLOGL A, SCHERER R et al. Graz-BCI: State of the art and clinical applications. *IEEE Transactions on Neural Systems and Rehabilitation Engineering* 2003:11(2), 1–4.

16. ZHONG M, LOTTE F, GIROLAMI M, LÉCUYER A. Classifying EEG for brain computer interfaces using Gaussian processes. *Pattern Recognition Letters* 2008:29(3), 354–359.

17. YOON JW, ROBERTS SJ, DYSON M, GAN JQ. Bayesian inference for an adaptive Ordered Probit model: An application to brain computer interfacing. *Neural Networks* 2011:247, 726–734.

18. Belmont Report. The Belmont Report: Ethical principles and guidelines for the protection of human subjects of research. http://www.hhs.gov/ohrp/humansubjects/guidance/belmont.html. Accessed January 14, 2015.

CHAPTER FOUR

Evoked potentials-based brain–computer interface

Abstract

Brain–computer interface (BCI) has a number of limitations, such as user fatigue and poor reliability, as discussed at the end of Chapter 2. Evoked potential-based techniques have been shown to overcome some of these limitations. This chapter introduces visual evoked potential (VEP) in electroencephalography (EEG) and describes methods to apply VEP for overcoming some of the limitations of BCI described in Chapter 2. The concept and implementation of steady-state VEP, along with the applications, user requirements, and limitations are described. At the end of this chapter, the current research activities in this area are discussed.

4.1 Introduction

BCI has been a trend in the communication between humans and machines. It probably uses the most direct way of access to the intentions of a person. A BCI system provides an entirely different output pathway and is the only way a person can communicate if the person suffers from disorders such as stroke, amyotrophic lateral sclerosis (ALS), brain or spinal cord injury, or any other diseases that can impair the function of the common output pathways. The disorders can impair the functions that are responsible for the control of muscles [1,2]. To overcome this disability, the electrical brainwaves of the person can be used to identify the action commands and to control machines and computers. These brainwaves are called EEG, and although these have been primarily used for clinical purposes, EEG is being considered for a number of control and interface applications. EEG signals can be noninvasively recorded by placing electrodes on the scalp of the person and amplifying the electrical potential. This recording is filtered and analyzed with suitable algorithms and classified to provide the user with the ability to communicate and directly control using their thoughts.

Currently BCI has been categorized based on the EEG brain activity patterns as follows:

- Thought-based BCI (explained in Chapter 3)
- Event-related desynchronization/synchronization (ERD/ERS) [3]
- Steady-state visual evoke potentials (SSVEP) [4–6]
- P300 component of event-related potentials (ERPs) [7]
- Slow cortical potentials (SCPs) [4]

Steady-state visual evoked potentials (SSEVPs) is the neurological phenomenon where VEP is used to identify the target of the vision of the person and is one of the event-related synchronized techniques. A VEP is an electrical potential that can be obtained from the scalp in response to a visual stimulus, such as a flash of light. There are different types of VEPs based on the stimulation frequency

- If the frequency is less than 3.5 Hz, the recorded VEPs are termed transient VEPs.
- If the frequency is greater than 3.5 Hz, the recorded VEPs are termed steady-state VEPs.

The concept of steady-state evoked potential is based on the brain responding to visual stimuli in terms of the phase and frequency of the stimulation. When a person stares at a stimuli, the parameters of the stimulation, phase, and frequency appear in the EEG recording. If there are multiple targets, each with a specific frequency or phase, the target that is the focus of the individual can be identified based on the analysis of EEG. However, the difference in the frequencies is small, and the EEG recordings consist of background brain wave activity, evoked potential, muscle activity, and noise.

In steady-state VEPs, the individual responses would overlap due to the presence of other signals and effect of multiple stimulation, resulting in a quasi-sinusoid oscillation with the same frequency as the stimulus [8,9]. The important step is to reliably detect this frequency with high accuracy and more important to detect when the frequency is not present, that is, the status when the person does not look at the stimulus. The later part becomes a very challenging task in BCI systems.

SSVEP has been used to control wheelchairs for those with disabilities. The user has to gaze at the icon or direction arrow, which gives visual flickering stimulation and the target is identified based on the frequency of the stimulus which can be extracted from the recorded EEG signal. The advantage of SSVEP-based BCI compared with other BCIs is that it does not require user training or calibration and achieves a high information transfer rate (ITR) [1]. It is easy to operate and configure, and is less susceptible to artifacts produced by eye blinks and eye movements because the EEG signal, recorded in the occipital area, is far from the source of such artifacts [10–12].

4.2 Brain–computer interface (BCI) systems based on steady-state visual evoke potential

SSVEP-based assistive devices have been developed to help people with severe disabilities [13–15]. They use naturally generated responses from localized brain sources as a result of visual stimulation, and translate the detected stimulus frequency into action. Although extensive research has been done in this area, but further work is still required to improve the practicality for real-world applications (outside the laboratory) and effectively interacting with the environment. This research has developed an SSVEP-based Speller BCI system and investigated some limitations of the available technologies as well as reporting the challenges and potential solutions to improve the system for real-world practical application.

The prototype speller system was built for investigation of optimum parameters affecting SSVEP response. The complete system consists of the four main parts:

1. EEG headset
2. Display/LED panel
3. Main controller/interface board
4. Processing unit

4.2.1 EEG headset

EEG was recorded wirelessly using the Emotiv EPOC neuro-headset (Research Edition) [12]. It features 14 EEG channels (10–20 international location system AF3, F7, F3, FC5, T7, P7, O1, O2, P8, T8, FC6, F4, F8, AF4) of 14 bit resolution (16 bit ADC with 2 bits discarded for instrumental noise floor) plus 2 CMS/DRL reference channels (P3 and P4). The headset is wirelessly communicating with a computer at 2.4 GHz band through a USB receiver. It also features wet electrodes and comes with special solution provided by the manufacturer. The device output is sequentially sampled at 128 SPS (2048 Hz internal) and the band limited between 0.2 and 45 Hz with two digital notch filters at 50 and 60 Hz. The headset is shown in Figure 4.1.

4.2.2 Display/ LED panel

The visual stimulator panel contained 40 arrays of 2 × 3 (2 rows, 3 column, 1 × 1 cm^2) white SMD LEDs (SMT 0603 super bright) each corresponding to a specific character, number, and/or a command (i.e., A–Z, 0, 1, …, 9, space, back space, Enter and Shift key) (Figure 4.2). All the characters were arranged in 8 (columns) × 5 (rows) cells with 4 cm intervals between LED arrays measured form their margin. The hardware configuration allows for independent triggering of each LED array at a specific frequency, which requires allocation of 40 different frequencies inside a narrow bandwidth. However, due to some other constraints, which will be discussed in Section 4.3, the maximum number of required frequencies was brought down to 8 and character detection was performed based on the interaction between SSVEP responses of columns and rows each trigged at specific frequency between 5 and 13 Hz. Each frequency was independently generated using a digital counter configured in an FPGA (Altera Cyclone II, EP2C5T144).

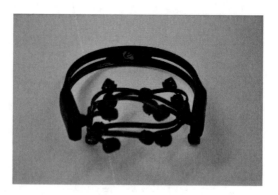

FIGURE 4.1   Emotiv EPOC EEG headset.

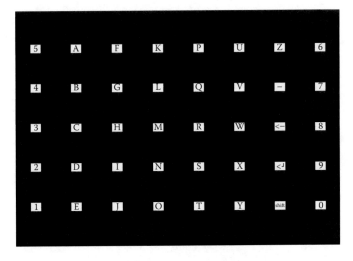

FIGURE 4.2   Speller LED panel (display).

Eight different counters corresponding to eight predefined frequencies were implemented. Each pulse was generated using an independent synchronous counter with 12 bits of resolution and zero phase angle. The hardware was equipped with a 50 MHz crystal oscillator as the reference clock and all the train pulses were produced using multiple divisions of the high frequency 50 MHz oscillator to obtain good frequency precision.

A multiplex-based subcircuit was also considered to switch between the columns and rows of the display panel when a command is received from the interface board. The block diagram of the implemented digital circuit is shown in Figure 4.3. According to this figure, the *clk_in* pin is the main clock input connected to the 50 MHz oscillator. The *Pulse_in* is the multiplexer's select pin, which is connected to the interface/controller board. The *Pulse_out* pin arrays are in the 40 bit vector each connected to an LED array.

4.2.3 Main controller/interface board

An interface circuit was built as the main controller for sending commands to the FPGA, initiating recordings, and switching on and off the stimuli. It was equipped with an 8 bit microcontroller (ATMega 8 AVR) and RS232 interface. The controller mainly is used as a communication interface between the LED panel and processing unit. The selection of columns and rows was possible through setting the Pulse_in pin to "1" and "0," respectively, based on the command received from

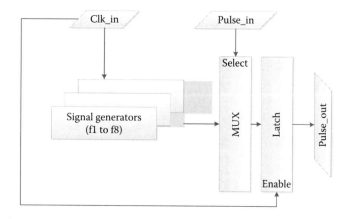

FIGURE 4.3 Block diagram of the implemented digital circuit: (a) the entire schematic, (b) the circuit inside the signal generator block.

the processing unit. The communication between the controller board and processing unit, which was a software package, was provided through a USB port and USB to RS232 converter module. The controller board and its different sections are shown in Figure 4.4.

4.2.4 Processing unit

A software package was written in Visual C++ 2010 express edition to (1) handle the recordings from Emotiv wireless USB receiver, (2) perform online signal processing, and (3) produce outputs by typing the characters on the screen. It was also equipped with a voice module to speak out each character that gets typed on the screen for user comfort and accuracy evaluation.

Mathematical operations and plotting were performed through integration of the MATLAB engine with the Visual

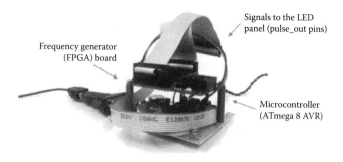

FIGURE 4.4 Main controller/interface board.

C++ platform and calling it from inside the platform. The software was also designed to send some instructions to the controller board via a separate USB port connected to a USB to RS232 convertor. The instructions included switching between vertical (columns) and horizontal (rows) lines of the display panel by sending "V" and "H" characters to the interface board.

Two different online signal processing algorithms were implemented and tested. The first algorithm was based on multivariable statistical canonical correlation analysis (CCA) in frequency domain in which two types of reference signals were used: (1) synthetically made sine and cosine expressions with different levels of additive Gaussian noise as reference; and (2) natural prerecorded EEG signals of the same patient as the training sets. The second tested method was based on implementation of a series of matched Gaussian filtering in the frequency domain and taking the maximum output SSVEP response for frequency detection. The detailed description of the latter, which had better performance, is as follows:

Among 14 available channels, 2 channels of O1 and O2 corresponding to Bain's visual cortex were used. A buffer of length 5×128 bits was implemented for each channel separately to keep the data for 5 s. The buffers were updated with 1 s intervals by shifting the old data 128 bits toward the most significant bit (MSB) and replacing the new samples in place of least significant bits (LSB). Signal processing was applied to the entire buffers within 1 s interval between the two updates. Each channel was treated separately until the very last stage, which will be explained later. At first, the data was normalized by dividing the entire buffers by its maximum value followed by autocorrelation operation.

The fast Fourier transform (FFT) was obtained and filtered with a band pass filter with 3 dB cutoff frequencies of 4 and 15 Hz. The reason for considering the filter bandwidth about 1 Hz wider than the used frequency range was to allow room for slight variations that may happen in the SSVEP response. A set of eight narrow band Gaussian filters were used to filter out each stimulating frequencies. The magnitude of each filter was set to 1 in order not to apply any gain factor. The mean values were set to center each filter at a specific frequency corresponding to the used stimuli (i.e., 6, 7, 8, 9, 10, 11, 12, and 13 Hz). The spreading factor σ of the filters was set to 0.5 to avoid overlapping with adjacent frequencies. Maximum output of each filter with known center frequency was buffered for later comparison providing 16 unique values (2 channels $\times$ 8 filters produced) every second.

The values of this buffer were sorted from maximum to minimum every 3 s (iterations) and center frequencies of the first three maxima were monitored. If the three frequencies were similar, the corresponding value was selected as the detected frequency. The process was repeated for each horizontal and vertical scanning, and the resulting two frequencies were obtained. As each character was encoded with two frequencies (one horizontal and one vertical), the detected value could be easily mapped to a corresponding character. A block diagram of the process is shown in Figure 4.5.

4.3 Design challenges and limitations

The design challenges and difficulties faced were mainly due to the limitation of Emotiv EEG headset and choice of this device for SSVEP-based BCI applications for the following reasons:

- Emotiv works only with wet electrodes soaked in saline solution. However, it is effective only for the first 20 min of the experiment and the pads will quickly become dry causing increase in the impedance and therefore affects signal quality.

- Emotiv comes with a test bench software to assist with correct electrode positioning and to ensure receiving the highest signal quality. However, this test only shows approximate locations inside a region of 1–2 cm. Slight displacement of O1 and O2 electrodes within that region resulted in different detection accuracies from no correct detection to accuracy of 90%.

- As a result of reaction between saline solution and metal bit of the electrodes, the pads and metal parts get easily molded, which affects the conduction path. The signal quality gets affected due to the grease and dirt in the pads when it is used for longer periods. Cleaning is required after it is used two to three times. The metal portion needs to be scraped with fine sand paper and the pads soaked in hot detergent water before it is used.

- The headset does not filter out high-frequency components due to any mechanical movement and tapping. Although it is equipped with a 50 and 60 Hz notch filter, the 50 Hz frequency appears in the spectrum of the raw signal with very high magnitude.

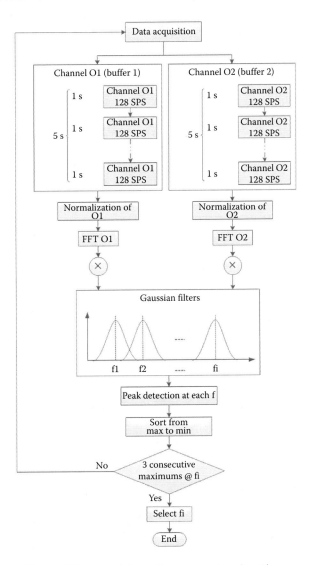

FIGURE 4.5   Diagram of the online processing algorithm.

4.4 **Results**

Figure 4.6 shows the spectrum of a sample EEG signal stimulated at 7 Hz after being passed through the Gaussian filter
series. According to this figure, the response from output of
the 7 Hz Gaussian filter has the highest peak value compared
to the ones from other filters showing that the stimulation had
a frequency of 7 Hz.

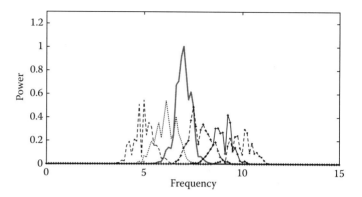

FIGURE 4.6 Output of the Gaussian filter series for channel O1 in the presence of 7 Hz stimulation.

Four subjects, three males and one female aged between 27 and 55, participated in the final test. The test was performed in a room with normal lighting condition (not in dimmed light). At first all the subjects were trained to use the speller system. The classification accuracy, *Acc*, was estimated based on the percentage of correct character detection among 10 trials.

The estimated time to output one symbol was 4.5 s/frequency (horizontal/vertical lines) and 8.5 s/symbol calculated as the average time for each correct output symbol plus the time required for switching between two characters (shifting gaze). The required 2 s rest was excluded from this calculation.

The experimental observations were

- In some subjects, like subject 1, one occipital channel was more dominant than the other in the sense that SSVEP response did not peak at some specific frequencies.

- The use of parietal channels (P1 and P2) for the purpose of Laplacian montage, which is defined as the difference between each occipital electrode and a weighted average of the surrounding electrodes (P7 and P8), did not contribute to any better classification accuracy; therefore channel P1 and P2 were removed from the processing to save computation time.

- The test on one subject was unsuccessful due to limitation of the headset. On this subject the headset signal quality check failed and did not detect a good-quality signal. This happened due to the subject's thick hair and a round head shape slightly larger than the average person.

- The classification accuracy of the system was 40% when tested on a subject (subject 3) with neuromuscular disorder and very thick hair resulting in poor signal quality for the O1 and O2 channels.

4.5 User benefits and improvements

There is a need for improvement in different areas for an SSVEP-based BCI to gain better classification results, which are as follows:

- Application of different scanning methods for more effective switching of columns and rows of the display LED arrays. Instead of triggering all the rows or columns at the same time, which will cause interference between SSVEP responses of the target frequency and the ones observed in the background due to impact of other adjacent stimuli, an approach similar to the scanning method used in matrix keypad boards can be taken. In this method only one column or row at a time will be switched on and flickered.

- This experiment showed that applying a 2–3 s delay between detection of each frequency can improve classification accuracy. This delay was applied for training the user to close his/her eye for 2 s before moving on to looking at another character; however, this could be implemented by turning off all the LEDs for 2–3 s after the detection of each frequency, then switching them back on.

- Emotiv has been very useful in demonstrating the functionality but needs further technical improvements to make it suitable for this application. This performed a radical paradigm shift of the earlier clinical EEG recording devices, which were very cumbersome and not suitable for being used outside a clinical setting. It has a number of advantages including aesthetics, cost, wireless capability, and ease of use. However, the signal quality is not stable and deteriorates over time and multiple usages. With Emotiv having demonstrated the possibility of such devices, we expect improved versions of such devices to be readily available soon.

- There needs to be an arrangement of frequencies, and different allocation order to columns and rows can impact on the output accuracy. At first allocation of frequencies to columns and rows was not in order to make sure that two consecutive frequencies do not appear next to each other. The reason was to keep the frequency distance between two adjacent columns and rows as large as possible to avoid any interference in the output SSVEP response and filtering problem. Therefore, for the eight columns the frequencies were ordered as 13, 9, 12, 8, 10, 7, 11, 6 Hz, respectively. However this resulted in lower SSVEP amplitudes for higher frequencies. When the patient stared at a frequency like 12 Hz, which is bounded between two lower frequencies (e.g., 9 and 8 Hz), SSVEP responses due to those lower ones were observed in the background and became comparable with the target stimulus frequency. Therefore, to overcome this issue the frequencies were arranged in the orderly manner as 13, 12, 11, 10, 9, 8, 7, 6 Hz.

- As one occipital channel may be dominant in some people, frequency allocation should be adaptive and modified for each subject, followed by the system training for the selected frequency range.

References

1. AMIRI S, RABBI A, AZINFAR L, FAZEL-REZAI R. A review of P300, SSVEP, and hybrid P300/SSVEP brain–computer interface systems. In *Brain-Computer Interface Systems—Recent Progress and Future Prospects*, edited by R Fazel-Rezai. 2013, pp. 195–213.
2. WOLPAW J, BIRBAUMER N, MCFARLAND D, PFURTSCHELLER G, VAUGHAN T. Brain-computer interfaces for communication and control. *Clinical Neurophysiology* 2002:113, 767–791.
3. PFURTSCHELLER G, LOPES DA SILVA FH. Event-related EEG/MEG synchronization and desynchronization: Basic principles. *Clinical Neurophysiology* 1999:110(11), 1842–1857.
4. ALLISON B, FALLER J, NEUPER CH. BCIs that use steady state visual evoked potentials or slow cortical potentials. In *Brain–Computer Interfaces: Principles and Practice,* edited by J Wolpaw and EW Wolpaw. Oxford University Press, 2012, pp. 241–250.
5. VIDAL JJ. Toward direct brain–computer communication. *Annual Review of Biophysics and Bioengineering* 1973:2, 157–180.
6. VIDAL JJ. Real-time detection of brain events in EEG. *Proceedings of the IEEE* 1977:65(5), 633–664.
7. SELLERS E, ARBEL Y, DONCHIN E. BCIs that use P300 event related potentials. In *Brain-Computer Interfaces:*

Principles and Practice, edited by J Wolpaw, EW Wolpaw. Oxford University Press, 2012.

8. DING J, SPERLING G, SRINIVASAN R. Attentional modulation of SSVEP power depends on the network tagged by the flicker frequency. *Cerebral Cortex* 2006:16(7), 1016–1029.

9. REGAN D. Steady-state evoked potentials. *Journal of Optical Society of America* 1977:67(11), 1475–1489.

10. SILBERSTEIN RB. Steady state visually evoked potential (SSVEP) topography in a graded working memory task. *International Journal of Psychophysiology* 2001:42(2), 219–232.

11. WU Z. Stimulator selection in SSVEP-based BCI. *Medical Engineering Physics* 2008:30(8), 1079–1088.

12. DUVINAGE M, CASTERMANS T, PETIEAU M, HOELLINGER T, CHERON G, DUTOIT T. Performance of the Emotiv Epoc headset for P300-based applications. *BioMedical Engineering OnLine* 2013:12, 56.

13. LIN YP, WANG Y, JUNG T-P. Assessing the feasibility of online SSVEP decoding in human walking using a consumer EEG headset. *Journal of Neuroengineering Rehabilitation* 2014:11, 119.

14. STAMPS K, HAMAM Y. Towards inexpensive BCI control for wheelchair navigation in the enabled environment—A hardware survey. *Brain Informatics* 2010:6334, 336–345.

15. YUE L, XIAO J, CAO T, WAN F, MAK PU, MAK P-I, VAI, M-I. Implementation of SSVEP based BCI with Emotiv EPOC. In *Proceedings of IEEE International Conference on Virtual Environments Human–Computer Interfaces and Measurement Systems (VECIMS)* 2012: 34–37.

CHAPTER FIVE

Myoelectric-based hand gesture recognition for human–computer interface applications

Abstract

Controlling a machine based on the myoelectric signal is very natural and is described as controlling the phantom hand for transradial amputee people using a powered prosthetic hand. This chapter introduces the technology associated with the recording and analysis of myoelectric signals, and describes the implementation of myoelectric-based human–computer interface (HCI). It then describes the limitations and challenges that exist due to the gross nature of the signal and presence of multiple muscle activities in the recordings. Finally, the current research activities that are identifying specific hand and finger movements and future directions in this field are described.

5.1 Introduction

Powered prosthetic hands are now commonly being controlled by surface electromyogram (sEMG) of the residual muscles of the stump. sEMG is the electrical recording of the muscle activity from the surface. It is closely related to the strength of muscle contraction, and an obvious choice for control of prostheses and other similar applications [1,2]. Several efforts have been made to identify commands from the stump of the hand, and for this purpose, two strategies have been considered: identifying individual finger movement, and identifying functional hand functions such as different grips. Each of these has their strengths and shortcomings.

Comparing the two strategies, identifying individual finger and grasp actions automatically by the machine facilitate the user of the prosthetic hand to control it naturally and allow for the maximum dexterity that the mechanical device can offer. But it suffers from shortcomings such as it does not provide the user with the ability to control the resting positioning of the finger and is sensitive to factors such as the initial location of the mechanical finger because it lacks the natural feedback to the user. For the device to be fully functional, it requires feedback to the user. Identifying functional grips have the advantage that they provide the user with the important hand actions, but suffer from the disadvantage that they do not allow the use of hand gestures for expressions and communication purposes.

5.2 Background

5.2.1 Identification of individual finger actions

Human hand actions result from the simultaneous contraction of multiple muscles. To accurately identify these actions requires determining the relative strengths of each of the associated muscles, and one method used for this purpose is to use an array of electrodes [2,3]. However, this requires significant equipment and is often unsuitable for being operated by an untrained lay user, and thus the actions are often estimated by using fewer channels of sEMG.

sEMG has the advantage of being easy to record noninvasively, and recent technical developments allow it to be recorded wirelessly, making it relatively nonintrusive. However, it lacks muscle selectivity and integrates the electrical activity from all adjoining muscles. A low level of muscle activity makes the signal susceptible to noise and artifacts. Different choices of global features of the signal using advanced signal processing and pattern recognition techniques do not address the fundamental issue and can at best result in marginal improvement. Although the systems reported in the literature are in general suitable for gross movements such as elbow flexion and extension, they are not suitable for complex movements where there are a number of muscles involved, and they have not been found accurate for wrist movements such as pronation and supination [1,2,4,5].

Some of the earlier attempts to identify individual finger actions were based on an estimate of the amplitude and the rate of change of the sEMG. More recently, the use of non-linear features, pattern recognition methods, autoregression (AR), and fuzzy clustering have been considered. Studies [6,7] have reported the improvements in algorithms in identifying the movements for myoelectric control systems. Tenore et al. [4,5] investigated the effectiveness of different configurations of array of electrodes (19 or 32) on the performance of the prosthetic control, both on able-bodied and transradial amputees.

Researchers have reported success in the use of multiple channels sEMG recording for controlling the prosthetic hand [4,8]. However, such systems are complex and the variation in electrode placement during sEMG recording can significantly vary the signal [9] making the technology unsuitable for being self-administered by the user or their caregiver. There is also significant intrasubject variation of sEMG magnitude between different experiments due to a number of factors [9]. A single channel system that can reliably identify the finger actions and in which the location of electrodes is not critical is highly desirable. However, overlapping muscles and the presence of noise and artifacts make this a challenging task.

Works by Smith et al. [10] and Xiang et al. [11] have attempted to minimize the number (six to eight) of electrodes to decode four different finger flexions. However, the number of electrodes is still very large. In an attempt to reduce the number of electrodes, Hope and Rassoulian used single-channel sEMG for determining the limb movement [7] using a predictive approach based on modular neural networks and reported 99% accuracy when tested on simple elbow flexion movement. Their system is cumulative and even a low error rate of 1% can result in very large error. The action of the finger is a result of the combined contraction of multiple muscles, and identifying the finger flexion requires determining the relative activity of the different associated muscles [12]. However, these appear to use black-box approaches, which attempt to identify small changes in the overall muscle activity in response to finger action, and this greatly limits the resolution, accuracy, and reliability.

To overcome the aforementioned shortcomings for low levels of muscle activity, the alternate method proposed by Plevin and Zazula [13] and Englehart et al. [14] is based on the decomposition of the signal into the fundamental components, the individual motor unit action potentials (MUAP). This is based on the knowledge that at very low levels of contraction, the MUAP are approximately orthogonal due very little overlap. One of the most progressive techniques for identifying MUAP at very low levels of contraction is the use of higher-order statistics and wavelets [14–16]. However, these techniques are based on the shape and estimate of the total density of MUAP, making them unsuitable when there are multiple muscles because the shape of MUAP from different muscles can be very different due to the difference in the transmission pathways [16].

Research studies are being conducted to improve the accuracy of the identification for better reliability and for controlling the assistive devices. Finger and hand grips are important functions for the disabled to interface with assistive devices such as prosthetic and robotic hands.

5.2.2 Identification of hand grips There are number of useful functional grip patterns that are achievable by the modern powered prosthetic hand. Grip patterns and maintained gestures are a result of complex combinations of contractions of multiple muscles in the forearm. It is important for the system to identify the desired grip pattern from the range of other grips and requires information associated with the strength of muscle contraction and the identification of the active muscles [7].

Various sets of features of the sEMG have been considered to identify the hand actions, such as the different types of grips. Since most hand grip patterns have only small differences in the muscle activity between them, the classification to identify the specific grip is challenging. This is even more challenging when the person has the forearm amputated because of the low signal level. Thus, the feature vectors of sEMG corresponding to these grip patterns are not sparse and have large variations in the distributions.

Grip patterns are more important for the disabled who are frail and have weak muscles to interact with the devices and control them independently. Due to computational complexity, currently there are limited devices/techniques which provide better reliability and accuracy in identifying the complex grip patterns such as pinch grip.

5.3 Current technologies and implementation

The techniques currently used are focused on identification of the following two groups of patterns: individual finger movements and finger/hand grip movements.

5.3.1 Individual finger movements Experiments were conducted with healthy and amputee participants to test and validate the technique to identify the finger movements [16]. Healthy participants performed the natural individual finger flexions. Prior to the recording, the participants were encouraged to familiarize themselves with the experimental protocol and with the equipment. For the experiment with the amputees, bilateral action training modality was performed, where the amputee participants performed the finger flexions with the healthy hand while performing the same flexion with the phantom limb [17].

The following specific finger flexions (as shown in Figure 5.1) were used for this study:

- Class 1: Flexion of little (pinkie) finger
- Class 2: Flexion of ring finger
- Class 3: Flexion of middle finger
- Class 4: Flexion of index finger

These generic actions were selected because they would allow the user to control individual fingers of the robotic/prosthetic hand. The participants performed the flexion without any resistance and were performed as was convenient and easily reproducible by the participant. sEMG was recorded when the participant maintained specific finger flexions. On-screen and oral command was given to the participant to perform the action and the order of the flexions was random. Each flexion was maintained for about 7–8 s during the isometric phase of the contraction when sEMG was recorded. The subjects were

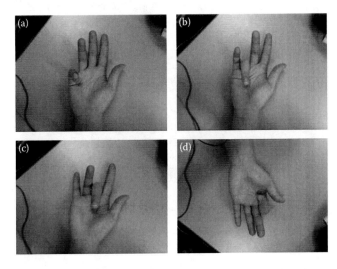

FIGURE 5.1 Different finger flexions: (a) Class 1, (b) Class 2, (c) Class 3, (d) Class 4.

given a rest period of 5 s between each action. Each flexion was repeated 12 times and the duration of each run of the experiment was about 120 s. The experiments were repeated on two different days to test the reliability and robustness.

5.3.1.1 Techniques to analyze the data

5.3.1.1.1 Preprocessing of the sEMG signal and removal of background activity   The first step of the method is to determine the temporal location of the MUAPs. For this purpose, the sEMG signal was decomposed using biorthogonal wavelet "bior3.3" and the wavelet maximas were identified [16]. This wavelet was chosen because it maintains the shape information and it has been experimentally found to exhibit the least Gibbs effect for this data [18].

The next step is the adaptive filtering of the background activity from sEMG. Wavelet maxima are obtained to locate the MUAP, and the magnitudes of the peaks (of wavelet maxima) are used to estimate the distance between the source muscle and the electrodes. The peaks are grouped into four groups in accordance with their magnitude and the relative densities of these groups determine the relative level of contraction of the associated muscles.

The recorded sEMG signal with the background activity is shown in Figure 5.2. Preliminary experiments indicated large variations in the background activity between different participants and between experiments. Spectral filtering, and thresholding, both, hard and soft, is unsuitable for such application because the noise characteristics are not known *a priori* [19]. For this purpose, an adaptive spectral subtraction technique was used to remove the background activity from the recorded signal.

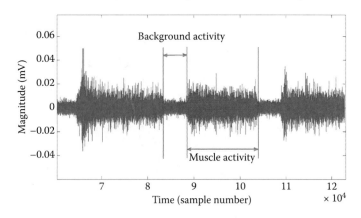

FIGURE 5.2   Sample raw EMG signal with background activity.

An adaptive filter was trained based on the background activity that was identified as the activity at the start of the experiments when all the fingers were relaxed and there was no action. The signal was filtered using wavelet bandpass filters using a 300 ms time window. The output was thresholded to generate a template and was subtracted from the recorded sEMG of the related experiment to remove the background activity.

5.3.1.1.2 Relative strength of contraction of the muscles After the signal was filtered using adaptive filtering, it was analyzed to obtain the location of the MUAP. The transients in the signal were located based on the location of the wavelet maxima [18] as in Equation 5.1. Only those wavelet maxima that were present in each of the scales and traveled from finest scale to coarsest scale were considered as corresponding to the pulse and the location of the MUAP [16,20]. Other wavelet maxima were rejected as random transients and is shown in Figure 5.4.

$$Wf(s, x_{n-1}) < Wf(s, x_n) > Wf(s, x_{n+1}) \qquad (5.1)$$

The relative strength of contraction was determined based on grouping the pulses based on the magnitude and determining the density of pulses in each group for the associated action. Cluster analysis of the preliminary studies demonstrated that there were four distinct magnitude ranges of the peaks for the four classes of finger actions. Thus, the peaks were divided into four groups based on the magnitude and density of each of these was obtained for each action. These four densities were the features of sEMG. These corresponded to the relative strength of contraction of the muscles. Thus, the analysis of single channel of sEMG gave a feature set consisting of four density of peak (DP) values, corresponding to the pulses belonging to four magnitude sets.

5.3.1.1.3 Classification The features of the single-channel sEMG were the input to the classifier, and the associated finger actions were the target. Twin support vector machine (twin SVM) linear kernel classifier [21] was used to classify the features. The advantage of using twin SVM is that it generates two separate hyperplanes and does not assume that patterns in each class arise from similar distributions. The system accuracy was validated using a tenfold cross-validation and tested using type I error (specificity) and type II error (sensitivity) [16].

5.3.1.2 Results   The average classification accuracy and the specificity and sensitivity for able-bodied subjects are reported in Table 5.1. The results have also been shown in the scatter plot (Figure 5.3). This plot shows the different clusters related to the different flexions. From Table 5.1, the overall accuracy of the detection of flexion of four classes of fingers (digits 2–5) was found to be 93.41% (±1.45) when sEMG was recorded from the distal end (experiment 1) of the flexor digitorum superficialis (FDS) muscle. It is also observed that there is a very small variation (1% decrease) in overall accuracy (92.4 ± 3.23%) when sEMG was recorded from the proximal end (experiment 2) of the FDS muscle.

5.3.1.2.1 Classification of data from amputee   The accuracy for identification of movements from the amputee has been listed in Table 5.2. The results show that the average accuracy of the detection of flexion of four classes of fingers (digits 2–5), which they performed based on the bilateral learning, was 81.87% (±13.54) from sEMG electrode location 2. The accuracy was found to be 74.59% (±12.52) from the sEMG electrode location 4.

5.3.1.2.2 Sensitivity and specificity analysis   The results indicate that the system specificity was high (~0.98) (range 0.96–0.99) leading to low type 1 error. The sensitivity of four classes was 0.94 (range 0.92–0.95) for experiment 1 and 0.93 (range 0.90–0.95) for experiment 2, demonstrating low type II error [16].

5.3.1.3 Discussion   The underlying principle of the technique is based on decomposing the signal to obtain the wavelet maxima that correspond to the action potential generated in the muscle. The magnitude of these peaks is inversely proportional to the distance between the muscle and the electrode site. The density of these peaks indicates the strength of contraction of the corresponding muscle. The combination of the range of magnitude and density of the peaks is indicative of the relative strength of contraction, and an indicator of the finger action.

During the training phase, analysis is performed and grouped into four magnitude-based groups. The method extracts the time-scale features, and identifies the wavelet maxima and the range of these maxima to characterize the signals based on the prior knowledge of the anatomy of the forearm. Recent studies did not demonstrate the level of contraction of muscle while the sEMG is recorded for classification. Dexterous finger movement control would essentially involve low-level

Table 5.1 Mean classification accuracy, sensitivity, and specificity of different classes recorded from distal end (Ch 1) and proximal end (Ch 2) from all subjects using the novel wavelet feature set

Class	Class 1		Class 2		Class 3		Class 4	
Channel	Ch 1	Ch 2	Ch 1	Ch 2	Ch 1	Ch 2	Ch 1	Ch 2
Mean	92.84	94.23	95.47	95.96	92.10	90.37	93.21	89.06
Amputee								
Mean	96.67	71.67	75.00	62.42	66.67	72.15	89.15	92.14
Sensitivity	0.92	0.98	0.95	0.97	0.92	0.98	0.93	0.98
Specificity	0.94	0.98	0.95	0.98	0.91	0.96	0.90	0.97

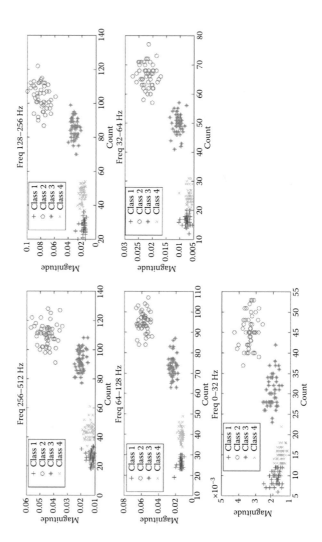

FIGURE 5.3   Scatter plot of features extracted from different flexions.

Table 5.2 Mean (±SD) recognition accuracy for the four grip patterns using twin SVM, LibSVM, and ANN

Subject	Twin SVM (RBF kernel)	LibSVM	ANN
Average (healthy)	89.11 ± 1.56	80.80 ± 1.22	78.11 ± 1.85
Amputee	78.25 ± 2.4	69.25 ± 2.5	65.25 ± 3.4
Sensitivity	0.94	0.90	0.92
Specificity	0.92	0.89	0.82

sEMG activity in active hand prosthesis. However, at low levels of contraction, signal-to-noise ratio is also low. This is due to background activity in the signal that adversely influences the quality of classification. This issue has not been addressed in any of the developed classification models. The technique developed in this study addressed this issue with empirically denoising the background activity. The clean signal obtained with this technique of noise cancellation provides better representation of the classes, even in low levels of contraction. This has also contributed to the high classification accuracy.

The results demonstrate that the technique was suitable for able-bodied people and was also tested for transradial amputee with good results. The results also show that the accuracy was not significantly affected by small change to the electrode location. It has also been demonstrated that the experiments were repeatable, with similar results obtained for experiments conducted on different days, even when the system was trained for only 1 day. This method has also been tested with the sEMG recorded from a transradial amputee. It would be desirable to reduce the number of electrodes to classify different classes because of limited available space on the forearm, especially in the case of amputees (Figure 5.4). For example, Touch Bionics' i-Limb (Touch Bionics Ltd., Scotland) uses only up to two electrodes for fine finger control, and systems employing a high number of electrodes may not be suitable for this kind of active hand prosthesis.

5.3.2 Hand/finger grip movements Recent studies have also investigated the fractal properties of sEMG [22,23]. Fractal dimension (FD) represents the scale invariant nonlinear property of the signal and is an index for describing the irregularity of a statistically stationary signal. It is a global and fundamental property of a system and should not be influenced by the regular changes within that system. Considering this criteria in the case of sEMG, FD should be

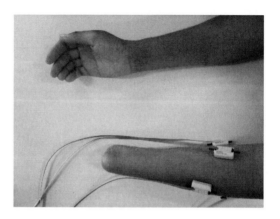

FIGURE 5.4   Placement of sensors for amputee subject.

the measure of the underlying system, which is based on the unchanging muscle properties [22]. Maximum fractal length (MFL), another fractal feature, is a measure of strength of muscle contraction [22], and previous studies have used a combination of FD and MFL to identify hand flexion [22,24].

Recent studies have used SVMs to improve the accuracy of classification. Multiclass classification problems are usually solved by solving many one-versus-rest binary classification tasks. These subtasks naturally involve unbalanced data sets. In the presence of unbalanced data sets, conventional error-minimization-based learning, as commonly employed in neural networks and SVMs, tends to favor the larger set, since we minimize the sum of errors across patterns. Although smaller class tests yield poor performance, the accuracy is good enough for practical use. The results demonstrate a striking improvement in classification results. Twin SVM also does not assume that patterns in each class arise from similar distributions. It allows the use of a different kernel for each class, which can be separately optimized based on the data. The facility for data-dependent kernel optimization for each class is particularly valuable in our application, and the results show that significant improvements can be obtained by exploiting this feature.

Effective use of twin SVM requires a multidimensional input vector [21]. This study has used a combination of fractal properties and features associated with strength of muscle contraction as the input to the twin SVM to overcome the previous shortcomings. Features such as root mean square (RMS), mean absolute value (MAV), and waveform length (WL) of sEMG have often been used as measures of the strength of the muscle activity and for identifying associated movements [25–27].

This study has used both the traditional features and fractal features to identify various grip patterns. We have used a combination of features that are associated with strength of muscle contraction (RMS, WL, and MAV) and the fractal features, which are associated with the muscle properties (FD and MFL) [28] to extract information from the EMG signal related to the grips. These features have been organized using three classifiers: neural networks, SVM, and twin SVM. Experiments were conducted on able-bodied and transradial amputee patients. The results demonstrate that the best results are obtained when features associated with the strength and the fractal properties of sEMG are classified using twin SVM.

5.3.2.1 Techniques to identify grip patterns

5.3.2.1.1 EMG recording procedures   Four bipolar electrodes (Delsys Inc., United States) were placed on the forearm of the able-bodied participants in accordance with standard procedures to record sEMG (Figure 5.5). These are active electrodes, with the preamplifier and two electrodes built into a single unit. The electrodes have two silver bars; each of 1 mm thickness, 10 mm length, and the fixed interelectrode distance of 10 mm. Electrolyte gel (Sigma) was used on the electrodes prior to affixing them on the skin [16]. The ground electrode was placed on the volar aspect of the wrist. For the amputee

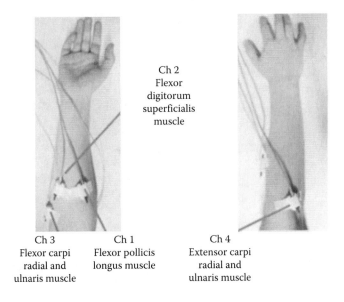

Ch 2
Flexor digitorum superficialis muscle

Ch 3
Flexor carpi radial and ulnaris muscle

Ch 1
Flexor pollicis longus muscle

Ch 4
Extensor carpi radial and ulnaris muscle

FIGURE 5.5   Placement of sensors for healthy subject.

participant, the electrodes were placed on the remaining stump of the participant as shown in Figure 5.4.

A labview-based sEMG acquisition system was used to record the signal. The sampling rate of the system was 1000 samples/s for each channel and the resolution were 16 bits/sample. Prior to the placement of electrodes, the skin of the participant was prepared by shaving (if required) and exfoliation to remove dead skin.

5.3.2.1.2 Experiments The experimental protocol was approved by the RMIT University Human Ethics Committee and performed in accordance with the Declaration of Helsinki 1975, as revised in 2004. Prior to the recording, the participants were encouraged to familiarize themselves with the experimental protocol and with the equipment. Experiments were conducted where the sEMG was recorded while the participants performed four sets of generic finger grip movements (Figure 5.6). These grip patterns represent the common functional grips required of the robotic/prosthetic hand.

- Grip pattern 1: All fingers closed together making a fist grip (Figure 5.6a)
- Grip pattern 2: Pointing grip (index finger pointing with other fingers and thumb closed) (Figure 5.6b)
- Grip pattern 3: Pinch grip (Figure 5.6c)
- Grip pattern 4: Holding grip (holding a drink can) (Figure 5.6d)

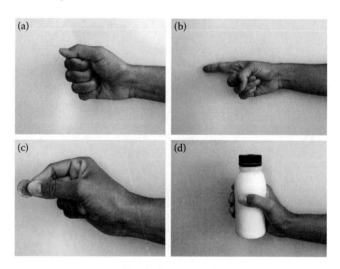

FIGURE 5.6   (a–d) Four generic grip patterns.

The able-bodied participants performed the flexion without any resistance and as was convenient and easily reproducible by them. sEMG was recorded through the experiment. The examiner gave on-screen and oral commands to the participant to perform the action without any fixed order of the fingers. Each flexion was maintained for 8 s and was repeated 12 times. The duration of each run of the experiment was 120 s.

5.3.2.1.3 Data analysis

The following features were computed [25]:

1. Root mean square (RMS)—RMS is the quadratic mean and is a statistical measure of the magnitude of a time varying signal and computed using Equation 5.2.

$$\text{RMS} = \sqrt{\frac{1}{N}\sum_{i=1}^{N} x_i^2} \qquad (5.2)$$

2. Mean absolute value (MAV)—The MAV of sEMG calculates the absolute value of data points and determines the mean of the resultant values based on Equation 5.3.

$$\text{MAV} = \frac{1}{S}\sum_{1}^{s} |f(s)| \qquad (5.3)$$

where S = window length; $f(s)$ = data within the window.

3. Fractal features—FD was calculated using the Higuchi algorithm [22] for nonperiodic and irregular time series. The first step for computing the MFL requires the computation of the length of the curve, X_k^m, for a time signal sampled at a fixed sampling rate, $x(n) = X(1), X(2), X(3), \ldots, X(N)$ as follows:

$$L_m(k) = \frac{1}{k}\left\{\left(\frac{1}{k}\sum_{i=1}^{\left[\frac{N-m}{k}\right]} |X(m+ik) - X(m+(i-1)\cdot k)|\right)\frac{N-1}{\left[\frac{N-m}{k}\right]\cdot k}\right\} \qquad (5.4)$$

where [ ] denotes the Gauss' notation and both k and m are integers. m = initial time; k = time interval; $i = 1$ to $[(N - m/k)]$.

The term $(N - 1/[(N - m)/k]) \times k$ represents the normalization factor for the curve length of subset time series. The length of the curve for the time interval k, $\langle L(k) \rangle$ is defined as the average value over k sets of $L_m(k)$. If $\langle L(k) \rangle \propto k^{-D}$, then the curve is fractal with the dimension D. MFL was determined from the plot as the average length $L(k)$ at the smallest scale and it represents the modified version of RMS and WL, as shown in Equation 5.5.

$$\text{MFL} = \log_{10} \left(\sqrt{\sum_{n=1}^{N-1} (x(n + 1) - x(n))^2} \right) \tag{5.5}$$

MFL is a recently established feature for measuring low-level muscle activation [22,23].

5.3.2.1.4 Twin SVM formulation Twin SVM, proposed by Jayadeva et al. [21], generates two nonparallel hyperplanes by solving two smaller sized quadratic programming problems (QPP) such that each hyperplane is closer to one class and as far as possible from the other. This is in contrast with the standard SVM formulation that solves a single QPP that has all data points in the constraints.

The twin SVM formulation involves solving the following set of QPPs:

$$\min_{w_1, b_1, q} \frac{1}{2} \| Aw_1 + e_1 b_1 \|^2 + c_1 e_2^T q,$$
$$\text{s.t.} \ -(Bw_1 + e_2 b_1) + q \geq e_2, \quad q \geq 0 \tag{5.6}$$

$$\min_{w_2, b_2, q} \frac{1}{2} \| Bw_2 + e_2 b_2 \|^2 + c_2 e_1^T q,$$
$$\text{s.t.} \ -(Aw_2 + e_1 b_2) + q \geq e_1, \quad q \geq 0. \tag{5.7}$$

where A is the matrix of feature points belonging to class 1; B is the matrix of feature points belonging to class 2; $c_1, c_2 > 0$ are parameters; e_1, e_2 are vectors of ones with appropriate dimensions; $w \in \Re^n$; $b \in \Re^n$; q denotes the error variable.

The twin SVM formulation based on generating nonparallel hyperplanes enables it to provide better separability for the features of the trials. The strategy of solving two smaller sized QPPs, rather than one large QPP, makes twin SVMs work faster than standard SVMs. The detailed explanation of the twin SVM classifiers can be found in Jayadeva et al. [21].

5.3.2.1.5 Classification   The four features—RMS, MAV, MFL, and FD—were the inputs to each classifier. The variations in the distribution of the feature vectors were removed by normalizing the data to zero mean to avoid the large interexperimental variation. Twin SVM, SVM, and ANN classifiers were tested. The proposed technique used twin SVM, using a one-versus-rest classification approach for multiclass classification with the radial basis function (RBF) kernel optimization technique. These feature vectors were then fed into the classifier. To compare, tenfold cross-validation was used to obtain the accuracy, sensitivity, and specificity for each classifier.

$$\text{Sensitivity} = \frac{\text{Number of correctly identified true class}}{\text{Number of true class}}$$

$$\text{Specificity} = \frac{\text{Number of rejected false class}}{\text{Number of false class}}$$

5.3.2.1.6 User requirements   This chapter has reported an HCI technique to identify four functional hand grips (and rest condition) by classifying the fractal features, RMS, and MAV of sEMG using a twin SVM classifier. The results indicate that when compared with other machine learning techniques such as neural networks and SVM, the twin SVM performed significantly better, with approximately 10% less error. Table 5.2 shows the classification accuracy of recognizing the grip patterns for various classifiers.

Twin SVM has the advantage over other classifiers that it uses a one-against-the-other approach, and determines multiple hyperplanes, each of which is optimized for each class. Such an approach overcomes the shortcoming of balancing between accuracy, sensitivity, and specificity. For the effective use of the prosthetic hand, sensitivity and specificity are two important factors. This is because poor sensitivity can lead to frustration for the user, while poor specificity results in erroneous functionality of the prosthetic hand and can lead to injury.

References

1. GUANGLIN L, SCHULTZ AE, KUIKEN TA. Quantifying pattern recognition–based myoelectric control of multifunctional transradial prostheses. *IEEE Transactions on Neural Systems and Rehabilitation Engineering* 2010:18(2), 185–192.

2. DALEY H, ENGLEHART K, HARGROVE L, KURUGANTI U. High density electromyography data of normally limbed and transradial amputee subjects for multifunction prosthetic control. *Journal of Electromyography and Kinesiology* 2012:22(3), 478–484.

3. TAO D, ZHANG H, WU Z, LI G. Real-time performance of textile electrodes in electromyogram pattern-recognition based prosthesis control. In *IEEE-EMBS International Conference on Biomedical and Health Informatics (BHI)* 2012: 487–490.

4. TENORE F, RAMOS A, FAHMY A, ACHARYA S, ETIENNE-CUMMINGS R, THAKOR NV. Decoding of individuated finger movements using surface electromyography. *IEEE Transactions on Biomedical Engineering* 2009:56(5), 1427–1434.

5. TENORE F, RAMOS A, FAHMY A, ACHARYA S, ETIENNE-CUMMINGS R, THAKOR NV. Towards the control of individual fingers of a prosthetic hand using surface EMG signals. In *Proceedings of the 29th Annual International Conference of the IEEE EMBS* 2007: 6145–6148.

6. HUDGINS B, PARKER P, SCOTT RN. A new strategy for multifunction myoelectric control. *IEEE Transactions on Biomedical Engineering* 1993:40(1), 82–94.

7. HOPE PW, RASSOULIAN H. Modular neural networks applied to surface EMG signals for limb function identification. In *IEEE International Conference on Systems, Man, and Cybernetics* 1999:2, 418–423.

8. CHAN FHY, YANG Y-S, LAM FK, ZHANG YT. Fuzzy EMG classification for prosthesis control. *IEEE Transactions on Rehabilitation Engineering* 2000:8(3), 305–311.

9. DELUCA CJ. Surface EMG; Detection and Recording, Available at: https://www.delsys.com/Attachments_pdf/WP_SEMGintro.pdf. Accessed on June 17, 2015.

10. SMITH JR, HUBERDEAU D, TENORE F, THAKOR NV. Real-time myoelectric decoding of individual finger movements for a virtual target task. In *Proceedings of 31st Annual International Conference of the IEEE EMBS* 2009: 2376–2379.

11. XIANG C, LANTZ V, KONG-QIAO W, ZHANG-YAN Z, XU Z, JI-HAI Y. Feasibility of building robust surface electromyography-based hand gesture interfaces. In *Proceedings of 31st Annual International Conference of the IEEE EMBS* 2009: 2983–2986.

12. NAIK G, KUMAR D, ARJUNAN S. Pattern classification of myo-electrical signal during different maximum voluntary contractions: A study using BSS techniques, *Measurement Science Review* 2010:10(1), 1–6.

13. PLEVIN E, ZAZULA D. Decomposition of surface EMG signals using non-linear LMS optimisation of higher order cumulants. In *Proceedings 15th IEEE Symposium on Computer Based Medical Systems* 2002: 4–7.

14. ENGLEHART K, HUDGINS B, PARKER PA. A wavelet-based continuous classification scheme for multifunction myoelectric control. *IEEE Transaction on Biomedical Engineering* 2001:48(3), 302–311.

15. KUMAR DK, PAH ND. Thresholding wavelet networks for signal classification. *International Journal of Wavelets, Multiresolution and Information Processing* 2003:1(3), 243–261.

16. KUMAR DK, ARJUNAN SP, SINGH VP. Towards identification of finger flexions using single channel surface electromyography—able bodied and amputee subjects. *Journal of Neuro Engineering and Rehabilitation* 2013:10, 50.

17. CASTELLINI S, GRUPPIONI E, DAVALLI A, SANDINI G. Fine detection of grasp force and posture by amputees via surface electromyography. *Journal of Physiology-Paris* 2009:103(3–5), 255–262.

18. MALLAT SG, ZHONG S. Wavelet transform maxima and multiscale edges. In: Ruskai MB, editor. Wavelets and their application, Boston: Johns and Bartlett, 1992. pp. 67–104.

19. ANDRADE AO, NASUTO S, KYBERD P, SWEENEY-REED CM, VAN KANIJN FR. EMG signal filtering based on empirical mode decomposition. *Biomedical Signal Processing and Control* 2006:1(1), 44–55.

20. ABEL EW, MENG H, FORSTER A, HOLDER D. Singularity characteristics of needle EMG IP signals. *IEEE Transactions on Biomedical Engineering* 2006:53(2), 219–225.

21. JAYADEVA J, KHEMCHANDANI RS, CHANDRA S. Twin support vector machines for pattern classification. *IEEE Transactions on Pattern Analysis and Machine Intelligence* 2007:29(5), 905–910.

22. ARJUNAN SP, KUMAR DK. Decoding subtle forearm flexions using fractal features of surface electromyogram from single and multiple sensors. *Journal of Neuro Engineering and Rehabilitation* 2010:7, 53.

23. PHINYOMARK A, PHUKPATTARANONT P, LIMSAKUL C. Fractal analysis features for weak and single-channel upper-limb EMG signals. *Expert Systems with Applications* 2012:39(12), 11156–11163.

24. ARJUNAN SP, KUMAR DK. Fractal properties of surface electromyogram for classification of low-level hand movements from single-channel forearm muscle activity. *Journal of Mechanics in Medicine and Biology* 2011:11(03), 581–590.

25. OSKOEI MA, HU H. Myoelectric control systems—A survey. *Biomedical Signal Processing and Control* 2007:13, 275–294.

26. KRYGER M, SCHULTZ AE, KUIKEN TA. Pattern recognition control of multifunction myoelectric prostheses by patients with congenital transradial limb defects: A preliminary study, *Prosthetics and Orthotics International* 2011:35, 395–401.

27. GRAUPE D, CLINE WK. Functional separation of SEMG signals via ARMA identification methods for prosthesis control purposes. *IEEE Transaction on Systems, Man, and Cybernetics* 1975:SMC-5(2), 252–259.

28. ARJUNAN SP, KUMAR DK. Fractal based modelling and analysis of electromyography (EMG) to identify subtle actions. In *29th Annual International Conference of the IEEE Engineering in Medicine and Biology Society* 2007: 1961–1964.

CHAPTER SIX

Video-based hand movement for human–computer interface

Abstract

The use of bioelectric signals has the disadvantage that users have to wear the electrodes on their body. This can be intrusive, uncomfortable, and not aesthetically pleasing. Such a device also suffers from being dependent on the ambient conditions such as temperature and humidity, and is sensitive to body sweat and movement artifacts, thus limiting the possible applications.

Recognition of commands from the video of the user has the advantage because recording the body movements do not require direct contact with the body and can generally be nonintrusive. This chapter discusses the technologies for recognizing hand gestures from videos and the challenges associated with the real-time implementations, and also describes an example of the implementation of the technology. The current research trend and future directions are also covered in this chapter.

6.1 Introduction

We perform actions with our hands to communicate with people and to control machines. However, disease or special situations can limit the ability of the user to effectively use their hands. In these situations, there is need for machine-based recognition of the hand actions or gestures. Such monitoring can be used for human–computer interface (HCI) electronic communication. Some of the many applications where these are used are facilitating people with acute weakness, computer games, telemedicine, virtual reality, and defense.

There are several ways to monitor the hand movement, and the choice of these is largely dependent on the applications and the ability of the user. These systems may be classified into two broad categories: (1) those that require the user to wear or hold some device and (2) video data. Some of the methods that have been considered for identifying the hand movement are the sensory glove, joystick, muscle electrical activity (electromyogram), and video analysis. Most of the current systems require the use of mechanical devices such as joysticks or gloves [1–3] or electrodes [4] that record the muscle activity.

Video-based techniques have the advantage that they are less intrusive and allow the free movement of the user. These are in two categories: those that require markers and those that do not. The markers that are used are either reflectors or clothing material that have special reflection properties. Most systems that are used for monitoring human movement require the use of markers. However, the use of markers is restrictive, and although they are less intrusive compared to the use of other sensors, markers do not allow the user natural freedom. The use of marker-less video monitoring is the most convenient method, but often suffers from limitations such as lighting and background conditions, and the computational complexity of video analysis that requires large computers and software.

This chapter provides a brief review of a marker-based system, and describes an example of a hand and gesture analysis method based on a marker-less system. In the subsequent sections, some historical examples and the limitations of each are discussed.

6.1.1 Hand-action recognition using marker-based video

Markers for video recordings are typically reflectors in the shape of disks that can be placed on different locations on the body. The other option is to use self-luminous disks. In both cases, these are easy to detect in the video or the image frames, and based on the prior knowledge of the anatomy, the movement of the body is determined. Most often the marker-based frames are converted using suitable software that connects between the different markers to depict the skeleton of the person, and the movement is easily viewed by the examiner. The software has the capability to measure different angles and rotate the image to view different planes. Such schemes are routinely used in gait laboratories or other human movement laboratories.

The design features and complexity of marker-based movement analysis can vary widely based on the application. Although some of these used for clinical lower limb examinations may use a large number of high-speed video cameras, applications such as for hand-action analysis may require only two cameras to provide three-dimensional movement information. For a detailed analysis of the hand actions, which includes the movement of the fingers and wrist, the system may require more than eight markers, and low-resolution, low-rate video cameras are sufficient. Researchers have shown that laptop-based camcorders are suitable for such analysis.

Marker-based video analysis of hand actions has the advantage that it is robust, and neither significantly affected by lighting and background conditions, nor by factors such as skin color. It also has the advantage of being suited for inexpensive cameras and software. However, the disadvantage is that it requires the user to wear the markers on their hands, making it unsuitable for a number of applications. It also requires the user to be in a specific region and plane, which can be highly restrictive.

6.1.2 Hand-action recognition using marker-less video approach

There are several devices that have been developed using video-based hand-action recognition. Fong et al. presented a virtual joystick technique based on static gestures to drive a remote vehicle [5], in which hand motions are tracked with a color and stereovision system. However, the system depends on the static gesture and does not recognize the action, thus limiting the applications. Baudel et al. developed a system called "Charade" to control remote objects using free-hand gestures [2]. Using Charade, a speaker giving a presentation can control remote computer display with free-hand gestures while still using gestures for communicating with audience. However, the system requires the use of data glove, and this limits the applications.

Another technique reported the combined use of video and electrical sensing and uses an "elastic graph," a conductive sensor, to classify hand postures against complex backgrounds in grayscale images [6]. But this technique requires the use of connected material on the user, and thus is not truly marker-less. Moy [7] and Bretzner et al. [8] have proposed visual interpretation of two-dimensional dynamic hand gestures in complex environments. It is used for humans to communicate and interact with a pet robot [7] and control home appliances [8]. The system is marker-less, but is sensitive to the background lighting and gesture positioning. Methods to improve this include the use of improved filtering to reduce the effect of the background, and hierarchical techniques to identify the actions in context [11]. Marker-less techniques are also sensitive to the difference between user skin color and texture. Number of methods to overcome this has been developed, and these can be classified into ones that require specific user training and the ones that are generic. One such method is based on the use of neural network developed for users and a mobile robot [12] interface.

An intuition-based system to provide naturalness suitable for two hands has been developed by Hummels et al. for computer-supported product design [13]. This interface supports perceptual motor skills and is task specific. A system that identifies user-specified hand actions and gestures is described in detail. This is a view-based approach for the representation and classification of predefined gestures using characteristics of the fine motion of hand gestures from a particular view direction using video data. The technique is based on the work of Bobick and Davis [12,13] and Sharma et al. [14] and uses a method called temporal history template (THT).

To identify the specific hand action from the THT obtained, the THT of multiple examples of the hand actions are obtained and these are represented by a set of features that are compact for the set of actions. The values of all the examples are combined and represent the specific action. Subsequently, the THT of the unknown action is generated and its features are classified to identify the closest match with the actions that were used to train the system.

There are several possible features that can be used for representing the THT and various techniques to classify the features to identify the action. In this chapter, the normalized centralized moments of wavelet subimages resulting from the decomposition of THT using stationary wavelet transform (SWT) has been used to represent the THT, and classification was performed using the K-nearest neighbor approach Mahalanobis distance [15–17]. This technique combines the use of geometrical centralized normalized moments and wavelet transforms, which is computationally inexpensive and is not sensitive to inter- and intrasubject variation of speed of movement. The results of classification accuracy of SWT with moment-based features are compared for the classification accuracy between the earlier works of authors for hand gesture classification of similar hand movements using Hu moments [18] and SWT with approximate wavelet subimages [19].

6.2 **Background**

6.2.1 Motion image estimation

For this work, a simple temporal difference of frame technique (DOF) has been adopted [15]. The approach of temporal differencing makes use of pixel difference between two or three consecutive frames in an image sequence to extract motion information [15]. The DOF technique subtracts the pixel intensities from each subsequent frame in the image sequence, thereby removing static elements in the images. Based on research reported in the literature, it can be stated that the actions and messages can be recognized by description of the appearance of motion [15–17,20–22] without reference to the underlying static images, or a full geometric reconstruction of the moving hand [23]. It can also be argued that the static images produced using THT based on the DOF represent features of time localized motion [15–17,20]. This process of generating the THT can be represented mathematically as follows.

Let $I(x, y, n)$ be the intensity of each pixel at location x, y in the nth frame. Then the DOF, $D(x, y, n)$ is

$$D(x,y,n) = |I(x,y,n) - I(x, y, n-1)| \tag{6.1}$$

The next step is the binarization of the DOF to obtain $B(x, y, n)$ over a threshold of Γ

$$B(x,y,n) = \begin{cases} 1 & \text{if } D(x,y,n) > \Gamma \\ 0 & \text{otherwise} \end{cases} \tag{6.2}$$

The next step is to incorporate a time function in this sequence. A ramp multiplier to represent time results in the generation of the THT where each pixel, $H_N(x, y)$ is a function of the time and represents the history of motion at that point. The result is a scalar-valued image where more recently moving pixels are brighter [15–17,20]. Consider the number of frames being considered for the action capture to be N. Then the THT pixels are $H_N(x, y)$

$$H_N(x,y) = \text{Max}\left\{ \bigcup_{n=1}^{N-1} B(x,y,n) * n \right\} \tag{6.3}$$

The THT grayscale images are then generated by temporal integration.

6.2.2 Wavelet transforms

The next step is the representation of the THT such that the representation is compact, while providing sufficient detail that allows the differentiation between different hand actions. Wavelets allow the flexibility because they offer multiresolution analysis, choice of a range of mother wavelet functions, and are also suitable for real-time analysis and thus are described next.

6.2.2.1 Wavelet The name *wavelet* represents the "baby wave" and as the name suggests is limited in time (for single-dimension signals) or space (for images). Unlike Fourier-based transforms that use wave functions that are of infinite length, wavelets are compact representations of signals. Wavelet transform of images have been found to represent the texture of the image at different levels of resolution.

Multiresolution analysis is achieved by using the mother wavelet, and a family of wavelets generated by translations and dilations of it. Dilation is the technique by which using the same function provides the resolution at different scales or frequencies, while translation is used for the wavelet to be used to cover the entire signal or image. A wide function can examine a large region of the signal and resolve the low frequency details accurately, whereas a short basis function can examine a small region of the signal to accurately resolve the time details [24,25]. For the purpose of this discussion, we will consider single-dimension wavelet analysis. If $\Psi(x)$ represents the mother wavelet, the scaling is accomplished by multiplying x by the scaling factor. If the scaling factor is a power of 2, this yields a dyadic series, such that the function becomes $\Psi(2^m x)$, where m is an integer. This results in a cascaded "octave band pass filter" structure.

If single-dimension time domain analysis is considered, the wavelet function Ψ is translated along the time axis to cover an entire signal. This translation is accomplished by considering all the integral shifts of Ψ

$$\Psi(2^m x - n)n \in Z$$

From this, the resultant wavelet representation of signal, $f(x)$, is

$$f(x) = \sum_{m} \sum_{n} c_{mn} \Psi_{mn}(x) = \Psi_{mn}(x) = 2^{m/2} \psi(2^{m/2} x - n)$$

$$(6.4)$$

where c_{mn} and Ψ_{mn} are the transform coefficients. These coefficients are computed by the wavelet transform, which is the inner product of the signal $f(x)$ with the basic functions $\Psi_{mn}(x)$. For classification, there is no need for computing inverse transform, since there is no need to reconstruct the original signal.

6.2.2.2 Discrete wavelet transform (DWT) The wavelet transform of any image can be successfully implemented by a pair of appropriately designed quadrature mirror filters (QMFs) [24,26–28]. Wavelet-based image decomposition can be viewed as a form of subband decomposition [24]. Each QMF pair consists of a low-pass filter (H) and a high-pass filter (G), which splits the signal's bandwidth into half. The impulse response of H and G are mirror images, and are related by

$$g = (-1)^{1-n} h_{1-n} \tag{6.5}$$

The impulse response of the forward and inverse transform QMFs, denoted by (~H, ~G) and (H, G), respectively, are related by $g_n = \sim g_{-n}$ and $h_n = \sim h_{-n}$.

For the purpose of image processing, a bidimensional wavelet is used. This can be understood as a one-dimensional, one along the x-axis and the other along the y-axis. In this way of applying convolution of low- and high-pass filters on the original data, the image can be decomposed in specific sets of coefficients at each level of decomposition.

Figure 6.1 shows the 2D DWT of image at level 1 of decomposition. The image is first filtered along the x direction, resulting in $f_l(x, y)$ and a high-pass image $f_h(x, y)$. As the bandwidth of $f_l(x, y)$ and $f_h(x, y)$ is half along the x direction, each of the filtered images can be down sampled in the x direction by 2 without loss of any information. The down-sampling is accomplished by dropping every other filtered value. Both $f_l(x, y)$ and $f_h(x, y)$ are filtered along the y-axis resulting in four subimages. Again the subimages are down-sampled by 2 along the y direction. According to the procedure, the image can be transformed into four subimages:

1. f_{ll} subimage—Both horizontal and vertical directions have low frequencies.

2. f_{lh} subimage—The horizontal direction has low frequencies and the vertical one has high frequencies.

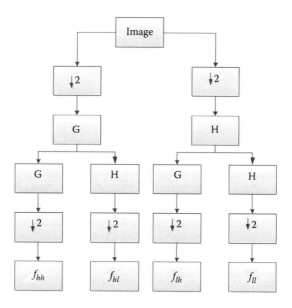

FIGURE 6.1 Multiresolution decomposition of image using discrete wavelet transform.

3. f_{hl} subimage—The horizontal direction has high frequencies and the vertical one has low frequencies.

4. f_{hh} subimage—Both horizontal and vertical directions have high frequencies.

6.2.2.3 Discrete stationary wavelet transform The classical DWT suffers from the drawback because it is unable to restore the translation invariance properties of the image. An alternate is SWT, which is similar to DWT and can be obtained by convolving the image with a low-pass filter (H) and a high-pass filter (G) but without down-sampling along the rows and columns [29]. Thus, the decomposed image is of the same size after decomposition ensuring the translational invariance (Figure 6.2).

Wavelet functions such as Daubechies (db), Haar, and Gabor are available at different lengths of the filter response. In this example, the "db1" wavelet was implemented [24].

6.2.3 Features of temporal history template (THT)   Hand gestures produce grayscale THT with global features and with variations due to the rotation and change in scale. Thus it is important to extract global features of the static image that are scale, translation, and rotation invariant. Geometrical normalized centralized moments are one such option of image

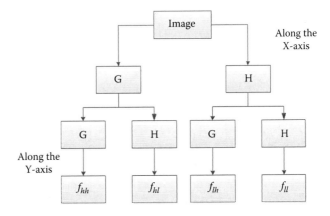

FIGURE 6.2   2D stationary wavelet transform of the template.

features and these are invariant to scale, rotation, and translation. The definition of the zeroth order geometric moment, m_{00}, of the image $f(x, y)$ is

$$m_{0,0} = \sum_{x=1}^{N}\sum_{y=1}^{M} f(x,y) \tag{6.6}$$

The two first-order moments, $\{m_{10}, m_{01}\}$, identify the center of mass (light intensity) of the object. This defines a unique location that may be used as a reference point to describe the position of the object within the field of view. The coordinates of the center of mass can be obtained based on the ratio of the moments

$$\overline{X} = \frac{m_{10}}{m_{00}}$$

$$\overline{Y} = \frac{m_{01}}{m_{00}}$$

According to uniqueness theory of moments for a digital image of size (N, M), the $(p + q)$th order moments m_{pq} are calculated for $p, q = 0,1,2\ldots$

$$m_{pq} \equiv \frac{1}{NM}\sum_{x=1}^{N}\sum_{y=1}^{M} f(x,y)x^{p}y^{q} \tag{6.7}$$

The centralized moments, μ_{pq}, of the image provides the translation invariance and can be calculated as

$$\mu_{pq} \equiv \frac{1}{NM} \sum_{x=1}^{N} \sum_{y=1}^{M} f(x,y)(x - \bar{x})^p (y - \bar{y})^q \qquad (6.8)$$

These centralized image moments are inherently translation independent but to achieve invariance with respect to orientation (rotation) and scale, these moments have to be normalized

$$n_{pq} = \frac{\mu_{pq}}{(\mu_{00})^\gamma} \qquad (6.9)$$

where $\gamma = (p + q)/2 + 1$ and $p + q \geq 2$.

6.2.3.1 Feature classification
For machine-based identification of the hand actions, the THT features have to be classified. There is natural variation in the repetition of the actions, and it is important to train the system to recognize the actions irrespective of the variability. There are several methods for classifying the system, such as the use of statistical measures, K-nearest neighbor (KNN) methods, neural networks, and support vector machines.

KNN-based classification has the advantage of being the simplest to implement and suitable for real-time applications. The first step in such a method is to develop templates of the features representing each action. Once the template representing the feature for an action is generated, the distance between the unknown action and the actions the system has been trained to identify is measured. When using the KNN method, the number of points that have to be considered is important.

6.2.3.2 Feature distance
To identify the unknown action requires comparing the features of the unknown action with the values of the actions the system is trained to identify. This requires the measurement of the distance between the features of the unknown and the various templates, and there are a number of distance measurement methods that are available such as Euclidean distance and Mahalanobis distance. This example has considered the use of Mahalanobis distance, which is a very useful way to determine the "similarity" of a set of values from an "unknown" sample to a set of values measured from a collection of "known" samples. It is computed by

$$r^2 \equiv (\mathbf{f} - \mathbf{k}_x)' \, \mathbf{C}^{-1}(\mathbf{f} - \mathbf{k}_x) \qquad\qquad (6.10)$$

where r is the Mahalanobis distance from the feature vector f to the mean vector $\mathbf{k}_x$, and $\mathbf{C}$ is the covariance matrix for $\mathbf{f}$.

6.2.3.2.1 Experiments to test the system   To test the efficacy of the technique, experiments were conducted where able-bodied volunteers were asked to make five predefined hand gestures (Figure 6.3) as follows:

1. Clasp
2. Move right
3. Move left
4. Hold
5. Grab

Each hand action was performed and recorded for duration of 3 s using a video camera located between 1 and 1.2 m from the hand at the sampling rate of 30 frames/s and in a well-furnished office environment. The video data was stored as true color (AVI files) and at low resolution with an array size of 120×160 for each recording.

6.3   Data analysis

The experiments resulted in a total 150 examples of the five hand actions. This data set was randomly divided into three subsets: training, validation, and test subsets. Half of the data was used for training purposes, and the other half was divided into two equal parts, such that one-fourth of the data was used for the validation set, and one-fourth for testing. Level 3–5 wavelet scales were found to be the most suitable for the analysis and were considered. The training data was used to develop the THT feature template for each of the five actions. The classification was performed using KNN and Mahalanobis distance. The results were tabulated to determine the confusion matrices for each action.

6.4   Discussion

Table 6.1 shows the movement identifier codes of different classes. Table 6.2 is the tabulation of the classification of the predefined hand movements using wavelets and geometrical centralized moments as feature vectors. The results of the

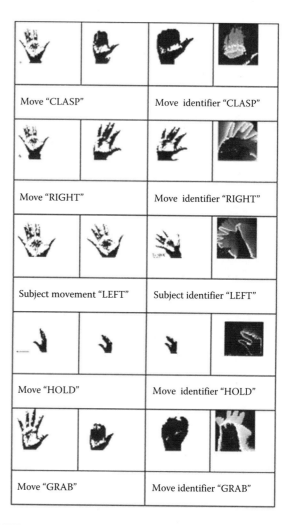

Move "CLASP"		Move identifier "CLASP"	
Move "RIGHT"		Move identifier "RIGHT"	
Subject movement "LEFT"		Subject identifier "LEFT"	
Move "HOLD"		Move identifier "HOLD"	
Move "GRAB"		Move identifier "GRAB"	

FIGURE 6.3 Representation of five pre-defined hand gestures.

testing showed that with the use of stationary 2D, SWT of grayscale THT to compute geometrical features, it is possible to classify the hand gesture classes with 97% classification accuracy. It is also observed that the classification based on the SWT with wavelet approximate images is time expensive [19] due to high dimensionality.

This work reported is with low dimensionality and is less expensive computationally with improved accuracy than reported by Sturman and Zeltzer [17] and Hu [20]. The results show an improved accuracy of classification when using SWT than when using Hu moments [20]. The results also demonstrate

Table 6.1 Movement identifier codes

S. No	Move description	Move identifier
1	MOVE "CLASP"	MC
2	MOVE "RIGHT"	MR
3	MOVE "LEFT"	ML
4	MOVE "HOLD"	MH
5	MOVE "GRAB"	MG

Table 6.2 Confusion matrix for classification data

Class	No. of actions	Predicted membership of classes					Accuracy (%)
		MC	MR	ML	MH	MG	
MC	50	47	—	—	—	1	94
MR	50	1	50	—	—	—	100
ML	50	—	—	49	2	—	98
MH	50	2	—	—	48	1	96
MG	50	—	—	—	—	48	96

improvement in classification accuracy and lesser computational expense as compared to the results by Kumar et al. [19]. The results also demonstrate that this technique overcomes intra- and intersubject variability. The use of wavelet transform to compute global image descriptors for image plane representation of THT makes the system less sensitive to small variations, and thus with better discriminating ability.

6.5 User requirements

The system is a stand-alone system where the machine can identify the hand actions of the user. The system uses minimum equipment and is computationally inexpensive, and does not require any other sensor or lighting condition. The major requirements for a system of this type are that the room has to be well lit, and the lighting and background conditions are stationary.

6.6 User benefits

Marker-less video analysis for hand-action recognition described in this chapter uses temporal history template of the action, and compares the template with the unknown using a set of geometric moments. The technique is robust and gives a high level of accuracy with very few false positives. The absence of any markers is a very desirable aspect of this method because it allows the user to have freedom without the constraints of any mechanical sensors, gloves, or the need for special clothing or even reflectors. The system uses a single low-cost, low-resolution camera and has been found to operate in the general office lighting conditions.

Such a system has a number of applications for able-bodied and disabled people. It can be used for controlling a computer such as during a lecture or presentation, or for playing interactive computer games. It may also be useful for machine-based e-communication where the computer can identify the hand gestures.

6.7 Shortcomings

Marker-less video analysis for hand-action recognition described earlier uses temporal history template of the action, and compares the template with the unknown using a set of geometric moments. Although the system has low error rate at 3%, this error makes it unsuitable for applications such as the control of a vehicle, wheelchair, or power machinery. This is because the error can be integrative and lead to major disaster if allowed to go unchecked.

6.8 Future developments

The use of video camera to identify specific hand actions has some untapped applications and significant potential that requires more research and development. Although this is a system that can be used in the current form, it is highly limiting because it only recognizes five hand actions. Another limitation is the ability of the system to work with only one hand. It is also limited because of the need for steady lighting and background conditions. New research is required to overcome these limitations.

One major opportunity to develop this technology further is to extend the ability of the system to work with both the hands, or when there are multiple hands in the frame such as when there are people sitting together. This will enhance the potential of the system and make it suitable for applications that identify the interaction between multiple people. The other development is to overcome the number of hand actions that the system can identify and significantly enhance this number. However, the biggest challenge is to overcome the need for steady background and lighting conditions. Overcoming this limitation will significantly enhance the application of this system. It is possible that this extension may require a hybrid system that uses marker-less and marker technology combined in one.

The possible extension of this technology can be beyond the hand actions and find applications such as for gait analysis. Such a system would be extremely useful for identifying the risk of falls among the elderly and for training athletes.

References

1. AKITA K. Image sequence analysis of real world human motion. *Pattern Recognition* 1984:17(1), 73–83.
2. BAUDEL T, BEAUDOUIN-LAFON M. Charade: Remote control of objects using free hand gestures. *Communications of ACM* 1993:36(7), 28–35.
3. POOLE E, KUMAR DK. Classification of EOG for human computer interface. In *Proceedings of IEEE EMBS,* 2002:1, 64–67.
4. MA N, KUMAR DK, PAH ND. Classification of hand direction using multi-channel electromyography by neural networks. *ANZIIS* 2001:PR106.
5. Fong TW, Conti F, Grange S, Baur C. Novel interfaces for remote driving: Gesture, haptic, and PDA. *Proc. SPIE 4195, Mobile Robots XV and Telemanipulator and Telepresence Technologies VII,* March 2, 2001: 300–311.
6. TRIESCH J, MALSBURG C. Robust classification of hand postures against complex backgrounds. In *10th IEEE International Conference and Workshops on Automatic Face and Gesture Recognition (FG)* 1996: 170–175.
7. MOY MC. Gesture-based interaction with a pet robot. *In Proceedings of 6th National Conference on Artificial Intelligence and 11th Conference on Innovative Applications of Artificial Intelligence* 1999: 628–633.
8. BRETZNER IL, LINDEBERG T, LENMAN YS. A prototype system for computer vision based human computer interaction. Technical Report ISRN KTH/NA/P-01/09-SE2001. Available at: ftp://ftp.nada.kth.se/CVAP/reports/cvap251.pdf. Accessed on June 18, 2015.
9. LAPTEV I, LINDEBERG T. Tracking of multistate hand models using particle filtering and a hierarchy of multi-scale image features. In *Proceedings of the Third International Conference on Scale-Space and Morphology in Computer Vision* 2001: 63–74.
10. BOEHME H-J. Neural architecture for gesture-based human-machine interaction. *International Gesture Workshop* 1997: 213–232.

11. HUMMELS C, SMETS G, OVERBEEKE K. An intuitive two-handed gestural interface for computer supported product design. *Gesture and Sign Language in Human-Computer Interaction* 1998:1371, 197–208.

12. BOBICK AF, DAVIS JW. Virtual PAT. A virtual personal aerobics trainer. In *Proceedings of Perceptual User Interfaces* November 1998: 13–18.

13. BOBICK AF, DAVIS JW. The recognition of human movements using temporal templates. *IEEE—Pattern Analysis and Machine Intelligence* 2001:23(3), 257–267.

14. SHARMA A, KUMAR DK, KUMAR S, MCLACHALAN N. Representation and classification of human movement using temporal templates and statistical measure of similarity. In *Workshop on Internet Telecommunications and Signal Processing* December 9–11, 2002, Wollongong, Australia.

15. DAVIS J, SHAH M. Visual gesture recognition. *Vision, Image and Signal Processing, IEE Proceedings* 1994:141(2), 101–106.

16. HINTON SS. Glove-talk: A neural network interface between a data-glove and a speech synthesiser. *IEEE Transactions on Neural Networks* 1993:4, 2–8.

17. STURMAN DJ, ZELTZER D. A survey of glove-based input. *Computer Graphics and Applications, IEEE* 1994:14(1), 30–39.

18. HU M-K. Visual pattern recognition by moment invariants. *IEEE—Pattern Transaction on Information Theory* 1962:8(2), 179–187.

19. KUMAR S, KUMAR DK, SHARMA A, MCLACHALAN N. Visual hand gestures classification using wavelets transform. *International Journal of Wavelets and Multiresolution Information Processing* 2003:1(4), 373–392.

20. KUMAR S, KUMAR DK, SHARMA A, MCLACHALAN N. Classification of visual hand gestures using difference of frames. In *Proceedings of International Conference on Imaging Science and Technology* 2002: 58–61.

21. PENTLAND IE. Coding, analysis, interpretation, and recognition of facial expressions. *IEEE Transactions on Pattern Analysis and Machine Intelligence* 1997:19(7), 757–763.

22. STARNER TP. Visual recognition of American sign language using hidden Markov models. In *Proceedings International Workshop on Automated Face and Gesture Recognition* 1995: 189–194.

23. LITTLE J, BOYD J. Describing motion for recognition. In *International Symposium on Computer Vision* 1995: 235–240

24. MALLAT S. A theory for multiresolution signal decomposition: The wavelet representation. *IEEE Transactions on Pattern Analysis and Machine Intelligence* 1989:11, 674–693.

25. DAUBCHEIS I. Orthonormal bases of compactly supported wavelets. *Communications on Pure and Applied Mathematics* 1998:41, 906–996.

26. SARLASHKAR ANB, MALKANI MJ. Feature extraction using wavelet transform for neural network based image classification. In *Proceedings of the Thirtieth Southeastern Symposium on System Theory* 1998: 412–416.

27. MALLAT S. *A Wavelet Tour of Signal Processing.* Academic Press, San Diego, 1998.
28. DAUBECHIES I. *Ten Lectures on Wavelets* (CBMS-NSF Regional Conference Series in Applied Mathematics, Book 61). SIAM: Society for Industrial and Applied Mathematics, Philadelphia, 1992.
29. CHUMSAMRONG WT, RANGSANSERI P. Wavelet-based texture analysis for SAR image classification. In *Proceedings of IEEE International Geosciences and Remote Sensing Symposium*, 1999:3, 1564–1566.

CHAPTER SEVEN

Human–computer interface based on electrooculography

Abstract

An electrooculogram is the electrical potential recorded from around the eyes and corresponds to the direction of the eye gaze. This chapter describes the signal and its properties, and the techniques to record and analyze the electrooculogram. It discusses the experimental results of the relationship between electrooculography (EOG) and the gaze of the eye, and describes a method to automatically determine the angle of eye gaze for controlling a computer mouse or a machine, and describes an example of the implementation of the technology. Consideration has been given to issues such as the reliability and the limitations of EOG for such applications along with possible solutions.

7.1 Introduction

Human–computer interfaces (HCIs) have a number of applications and can have different impacts on many individuals. For some, it opens the world of virtual reality and the control of machinery without physical contact, while for others it means increased independence from disabilities. Researchers have developed many systems to facilitate man–machine interfaces, and one important modality is the use of eye gaze. There are a number of assistive applications where detecting the eye gaze is useful for controlling a computer or peripheral devices. Such devices can play a role in helping people with disabilities who do have eye gaze control but have lost the effective use of their hands. Other applications include the use of gaze-controlled weapon control for defense personnel. Another application of eye movement identification is for sleep-related research, where eye movement is indicative of the type of sleep.

Eye-gaze detection techniques can use invasive and noninvasive methods. Assistive technology applications generally use noninvasive and minimum intrusive systems. There are two major noninvasive techniques used to identify the gaze of an individual and these are based on two modalities: camera and electrical activity. The camera-based system identifies the location of the two eyes and estimates the direction of the gaze, while the use of electrical activity recorded around the eye, referred to as EOG, measures the eye gaze from the electrical potential. In this chapter, the EOG-based HCI is discussed.

7.2 Background

7.2.1 Eye movement

Most humans are easily able to follow the visual path of a moving object. This may involve the combination of head and eye movement. Detecting the eye movement when it is following a path has a number of medical and nonmedical applications and can be achieved using the corresponding bioelectric signals recorded. There are various applications where detecting eye movement and eye-gaze direction is important. These applications can be broadly categorized as

- Virtual reality
- Computer games
- Medical diagnostics
- Assistive technology for disabled
- Advertising research

The sensing, detection, and consequent analysis of eye movement and the direction of eye gaze has found applications for assistive technologies and other fields such as virtual reality, computer games, and defense. Different applications require different features, and there are a number of techniques that have been developed. The methods for detection of eye movement can be invasive and noninvasive [1], where the invasive methods require the placement of some part of the detection system in the eye. Some of the different methods that are currently available are listed in Table 7.1.

Table 7.1   Eye movement detection methods

Category	Detection type	Description
Invasive (contact type)	Optical lever	Reflection from contact lens measured by a photoelectric device
	Search coil	Contact containing a magnetic coil, inserted onto the sclera of the eye, a magnetic field induces a voltage in a coil
Noninvasive (noncontact type)		Trained observer estimates movement
		Video, still frames; software analysis or by hand
	Infrared reflection	Photo cell detects reflectance of the infrared source from the surface of the eye
	Electrooculography	Electrodes placed on skin, pick up corneal-retinal potential

Each of the aforementioned techniques have their own strengths and thus are most suitable for specific applications. Some of the important attributes that have been identified in the literature that allow a comparison and matching of most of the techniques with the application are

- *Spatial resolution*—In image processing, spatial resolution is a measure of the distance between two objects that can be distinguished. Similarly, in HCI, this is a measure of the distance between two gaze angles that can be separately distinguished. Depending on the application, the minimum resolution required could be different. In some detection methods (video, infrared) software is used to determine the spatial reference point from data. In these methods, it is not as important that the recorded data is accurate as long as there is a known reference point.

- *Temporal resolution*—The maximum rate of change of the angle of the gaze that the system can recognize is the temporal resolution. Some applications where the saccadic movement has to be recognized may require significantly higher temporal resolution, where eye movements corresponding to 700 degree/s may be important.

- *Vertical and horizontal movement*—There is a distinct difference between the human eye control and movement in horizontal and vertical movements. There are many applications where the emphasis is on the horizontal movement, and there are others where both the vertical and horizontal movements are relevant. Such systems can also have the added complexity of eye blink movement.

- *Setup time*—Setup time indicates the time required for preliminary setup of the device for the user, required calibration, and testing. The various modalities have significant differences in the time required to set up the system for the user. Depending on the application the maximum acceptable setup time may be different and thus would limit the choice of modality.

- *Cost*—There can be significant differences in the cost of the different systems, and while some applications may absorb higher costs, there would be other systems that are cost-sensitive. A system that has high cost restricts the use and availability of the system.

Although there are a number of methods to detect eye movement, not all are suitable for a control system implementation. It is for this reason that there have been a greater number of practical control systems implementing EOG as a preferred method of detecting eye movement.

7.2.2 Electro-oculography (EOG)

EOG is the recording of the corneal–retinal potential (dipole) of the eye, the potential that exists between the front and the back of the eye [2,3]. As the eye moves in either the transverse or the vertical plane, the positive and negative poles of the dipole move closer to the respective electrode changing the potential that the electrode records. The principal is illustrated in Figure 7.2. Identification of the movement of the eye, the number of electrodes, and thus the complexity may vary. Depending on the required application, as little as one set of differential electrodes (two electrodes) or as many as eight electrodes, plus a commons, may be used to record the electrooculogram.

To measure eye movement, pairs of electrodes in a differential mode are placed across the eye, either above and below the eye or to the left and right of the eye. A reference electrode is typically placed at a farther point, such as the ear. When the eye moves away from the center toward the side, it moves closer to one of the two electrodes and farther from the other. Thus, the

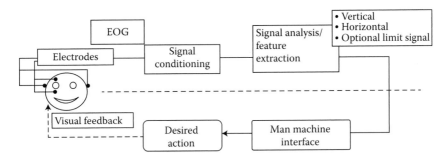

FIGURE 7.1 Basic EOG control system.

electrode that the eye moves closer to, becomes more positive while the opposite electrode becomes negative. Consequently, a potential difference occurs between the two electrodes. If the resting potential is constant, the recorded potential is a measure of the eye's position. For example, when the person gazes left, the cornea approaches the electrode near the outer canthus of the left eye, resulting in this electrode having a positive potential, and the right gaze will lead to the opposite.

Systems that use EOG, detect the direction of an individual's gaze, and from the biosignals recorded, the HCI determines a set of spatial angles of the eye gaze. This is combined with the screen information to generate control command signals that are then applied to enact the required action. A simplified system is shown in Figure 7.1.

In this chapter, the relationship between different aspects of eye movement and EOG has been described and EOG signal-based assistive device applications are investigated. An EOG-based system is described and the experimentally obtained relationship between EOG and eye gaze is shown.

The investigation acquired EOG data from various test subjects while they fixated their gaze on fixed and moving target points. Specific features of the recorded electrooculogram were extracted during preliminary analysis to assist with the selection of a method to generate spatial controls. Additional investigations of the collected data have assisted with determining the feasibility of recognizing the angular displacements and generating an output that is representative of the required movement.

7.2.3 Human eye anatomy: Movement

The human eye has six muscles and requires two or more of these muscles for eye movement or fixation. These six muscles enable movement in the transverse, longitudinal (torsional), and vertical directions; their respective attachment locations on the eye can be seen in Figure 7.2. An explanation of the actions performed

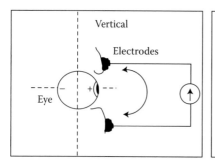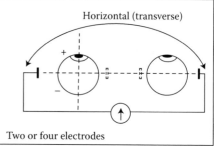

FIGURE 7.2   Placement of electrodes to record electrooculogram signals.

by the six muscles can be found in many physiology texts [4,5]. It has also been reported that the movement of a specific pair of eye muscles is antagonistic when the eye moves, allowing an excellent degree of motion control. The directions in which each pair of muscles moves the eye are detailed in Table 7.2.

It has also been reported that human eyes cannot move independently in the vertical direction (nonconjugate movement). This restriction may cause limitations in some systems, which record the vertical eye movement of an individual, but in general, has the advantage that it reduces the complexity of some noninvasive systems such as EOG.

EOG was first discovered around 1920 by placing two electrodes on the skin around the eye. It was observed that one could record electrical activity that changed in synchrony with movements of the eye. At that time, this was considered to be because of the muscle activity, the action potentials in the muscles that are responsible for moving the eyes in the orbit. However, it was later found that this electrical potential is due to the permanent potential difference that exists between the front and the back of the eye, the cornea, and ocular fundus potential, which is approximately 30 mV, the front of the eye being positive.

Table 7.2   Action of muscles of the human eye

Muscles	Actions
Medial rectus, lateral rectus	Horizontal (left, right)
Superior rectus, inferior rectus	Vertical (up, down)
Superior oblique, inferior oblique	Torsional around the longitudinal axis

7.3 Current technologies: Historical to state of the art

One of the early examples of eye-gaze-based assistive technology was "EagleEyes." This system was first developed and reported in 1996 [6]. It was designed to assist individuals with disabilities to communicate or control devices. EagleEyes was designed to facilitate the users to initiate actions or communicate with their personal computer interface simply by moving their eyes to fixate on a specific location on a monitor. The system applied four electrodes for vertical and horizontal movements and custom-designed software for the determination of the coordinates of the cursor on the PC monitor. The system allowed the user to move the cursor around a screen by moving the fixation point (gaze) of their eyes. The software also included an option that sensed the duration of the stare, and using this variable could identify the user command. Identification could also be replaced by using the eye blink, though that may significantly slow the system.

The EagleEyes system was tested on able-bodied individuals and the users could select letters on the screen to perform tasks such as spelling of their names on a PC monitor and for this they required very little training. It was also tested for individuals with disabilities and was found to be suitable for them, but required significantly more training when being used by people suffering disabilities. The software for PC screen display was a significant improvement to other displays of the mid-1990s, and there were options of multiple displays for text and graphics that the individual could select. Thus, it enabled the user to interact and access Internet resources only using their eye gaze. Since the original system was first reported, several variants and improvements have been developed.

Assistive technology applications of EOG are not just limited to the controlling of a cursor on a PC monitor, but include the control of devices such as a wheelchair or a car. Over the past three decades, researchers have developed wheelchair systems that can accept direction commands from an EOG-based system [7]. One such system has been designed to analyze the electrooculogram signals using a neural network. The signals from the two horizontal electrodes and two vertical electrodes are analyzed by software installed on a laptop that is integrated with the chair.

EOG systems require the fixation of the head, which is uncomfortable when the device has to be used on a regular basis. Thus, the common limitation of EOG systems is that these determine the angle of the gaze with respect to the head of the individual. To overcome this limitation, the head movement has to be determined to obtain the absolute angle of the gaze and thus the object being gazed by the user. The other requirement of the system is to include a trigger mechanism for which the person can indicate the gaze selection. There are a number of options to track head movement and to obtain the trigger command. These are described next.

One inexpensive, portable, and reliable way to measure head movement is to use an electromagnetic tracking device [8]. Such a system can be integrated within a cap of the user that detects the relative angle of the head with respect to the predefined axis. Integrating the measure of the angle of the head along with EOG can determine the object being gazed by the user and allows the user the freedom to move their head normally.

In early systems the head was stationary and the eyes moved, while in the new system the spatial movement of the individual's head is determined by analysis of a magnetic field from a transmitter attached to the head. Receivers that have been located at specific locations around the individual detect the magnetic field, enabling the spatial movement of the head to be determined. The system was found to improve the freedom of head movement without unduly affecting the system accuracy.

A further application has used the electrooculogram signal from the eyes to mimic a PC mouse [9]. Vertical and horizontal movements are recorded. The motion of a serial-type mouse and its controls were duplicated by the individual's eye movement and blinking, with two and three blinks being reported to correspond to single and double mouse clicks. The system moved the cursor when it was determined that the eyes had moved greater than a defined angle. The cursor remained moving along the detected direction until two blinks, separated by a specific time interval, were detected at which point it stopped. During practical testing, the system was found to function as required.

One of the shortcomings of EOG-based systems was the need for wires. The system required wires hanging in the face of the user, which limits the possible applications and is not aesthetically pleasing. The wires can also result in movement artifacts and lead to poor signal quality. To overcome this shortcoming, EOG-based mouse control systems with wireless links were developed and reported by Norris and Wilson [10]. This system used a novel approach for electrode placement using four electrodes, each attached to a pair of spectacles. The electrodes were connected using a combination of wired and wireless connectivity such that there were no visible wires. The advantage of such a system is the convenience, aesthetics, non-intrusive nature of such electrodes, and improved reliability. In such a system, two electrodes were located near the outer edge of each eye, while the other two were located on the bridge of the nose. The eye blink was separated from EOG based on the frequency filter banks, with eye blink corresponding to the lower frequency.

The aforementioned work reports the identification of the signature of vertical and horizontal eye movements from the signal that was achieved by training the system for the individual user. A virtual lead was generated using the recordings for estimating the vertical movement and this was obtained from the training of the data to targeted movement.

One difficulty with these systems is that these identify the angle of the gaze and thus identification of the object being gazed is obtained by superimposing the two discrete information: angle of gaze and the screen display. This system has drawbacks and is not natural as we view our environment in three dimensions; the aforementioned systems reduce the information to two dimensions. To overcome this, the system that improved the earlier techniques [11] developed an interface with the capability to determine the 2D and 3D fixation points. The system was designed to operate with a 19-inch monitor that displays a series of selection boxes separated by 3 degrees. The system also has the capability for the inclusion of additional options that would allow eye blinks and other facial gestures to be recognized as legitimate actions. The system has also been reported to function successfully.

7.3.1 System requirements

An electrooculogram is a low-frequency, low-voltage electrical recording and is recorded using purpose-built differential amplifiers. Filters are required to remove artifacts due to movement of electrodes, electromyograph, and line noise. For this purpose, the signal has to be recorded using two channels of differential amplifiers with the typical gain being around 500–2000 differential gain. To reduce the noise, the amplifier should have high common-mode rejection ratio (CMRR), such as being greater than 90.

All systems reported that they filtered the EOG signals using high-pass and low-pass filters to restrict the effects of drift and influences of other artifacts such as changes to electrode adhesion, electromyograph signals, and electroencephalograph signals. The filter 3 dB bandwidths were generally 0.16 Hz for high-pass filters and between 15 and 20 Hz for the low-pass filters. In several systems it has been indicated that the direct current (DC) restoration level is established to counter the effects of DC drift.

EOG requires the use of surface electrodes. There are a number of different electrodes that are available. The use of Ag/AgCl is useful because such electrodes are more stable and there are less movement artifacts. The anatomy of the face permits only the use of self-adhesive type of electrodes, and thus many of the general-purpose Ag/AgCl self-adhesive electrodes may be used. These electrodes are disposable and generally inexpensive. If the electrodes being used are dry, adding suitable nonflowing, highly ionic gel is desirable.

Cleaning the skin prior to applying the electrodes is essential to ensure good contact and thus lower noise. Poor contact between the electrodes and the skin can result in line noise such that 50 or 60 Hz (based on what is the power frequency) will be recorded alongside the electrooculogram and can result in very poor analysis.

7.4 Example of EOG-based system

7.4.1 Introduction

The electrooculogram is the standing potential of the eye and is a product of the dipole that is formed by the cornea and the retina, and is mainly a function of the angular displacement of the eye in the eye socket. The design and test methodology of the current study has been formulated assuming that the electrooculogram is entirely a function of the angular displacement of the eye in its socket. In this example, the electrooculogram has also been assumed to be independent of the differences between people such as distance of a specific target from the eye and possible physiological anomalies.

It is also been assumed that the distance between the object and the eye, or the depth, is not going to change the electrooculogram. This rationale has led to the test environment being modeled as a series of target points in 3D space. Each target point exists on the surface of a sphere with the human subject effectively positioned at the center of the sphere. The coordinates of the subject's eyes are located at a specific measurable height above the origin of the sphere. The spatial orientation of the subject's eyes as they fixate on a specific target point can therefore be determined using the detected electrooculogram.

7.4.2 System description

Based on the assumption that the measured electrooculogram is independent of the distance between the object and the user, a series of target points were attached to vertical and rigid posts positioned on the circumference of a circle of known radius. Each target was located 15° apart relative to the *x*-axis obtained (arbitrarily) from the center of the circle, with the target points at the extremes being located at 60° either side of a target point nominated as the reference target. This gave nine target points in the horizontal plane, as shown in Figure 7.3.

For the horizontal plane all targets were positioned to be at approximately eye height when test subjects were seated, although this was not considered critical to the accuracy of the recorded electrooculogram in the horizontal plane. Minor variations in the height of the target relative to the eye height of the test subject would tend to affect only the vertical electrooculogram recorded, which in theory would remain at 0° during the specific horizontal testing phase.

The reference target point was positioned directly in front of the test subject's eyes, at a measured eye height, allowing a known starting point for all electrooculogram measurements in the horizontal plane. The location of the reference point also ensured that there would be minimal inclination or declination of the eyes in the vertical plane and minimal angular offset of the eyes in the horizontal plane, when test subjects were instructed to fixate their eyes (gaze) on the reference point.

To determine the relationship of electrooculograms corresponding to the movement of the eye in the vertical plane, test points were attached to the reference pole. Test points were positioned to give five equally spaced sections between 45° above the eye level and the target point at the floor level, below

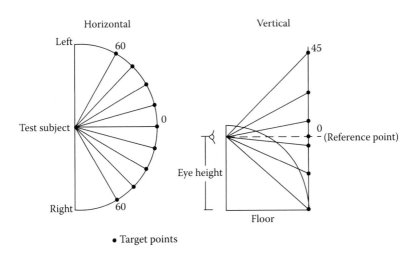

FIGURE 7.3 Configurations of targets.

the reference pole. The positions of the vertical target points are shown schematically in Figure 7.5.

To reduce interexperimental and intersubject variability and maintain commonality of test target angles from one test subject to another, the subjects were seated such that the height of their eyes (from the floor) was similar. For the current investigation, four test subjects had their eye height set at 1.3 m and one subject at 1.2 m. The changes in vertical angles during eye movement were determined based on the trigonometric relationship between the distances. It was assumed that eye movement is not simultaneous in both horizontal and vertical planes and thus there would be minimal electrooculogram eye movement recorded in the orthogonal plane.

7.4.3 Experimental protocol

Electrooculogram signals were recorded from five subjects, consisting of four males and one female. The eye physiology of each subject was not considered for this investigation and therefore any effects can only be surmised.

Five disposable, self-adhesive Ag/AgCl universal electrodes (Nessler Med–Technin, Austria, Ref 1066) were placed around the eyes as shown in Figure 7.4. Two electrodes were attached to the outer canthi of each eye and formed a differential electrode pair for horizontal movement. Two electrodes were placed above and below the right eye to form a differential electrode pair for vertical movement. A fifth electrode was placed at the center of the forehead as a common ground. Prior to the attachment of the electrodes, the skin was cleaned and wiped using a rough facial paper.

The signals were sampled at 1000 Hz with an internal anti-aliasing filter cut-off frequency set at 500 Hz and alternating

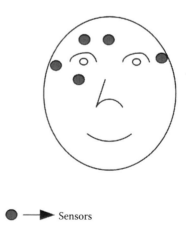

● ⟶ Sensors

FIGURE 7.4   Placement of electrodes on test subject.

current (AC)-coupled amplifiers with a time constant, T_c, of 15 s. The time constant entered effectively gave a 0.011 Hz high-pass filter and this dictated that prior to recording any data, a period of $5 \times T_c$ (25 s) pass. This time was required to allow the system to reach a steady-state level after the commencement of data recording.

7.4.4 Experimental procedure

As a first step, the integrity of the acquisition system was checked. Prior to recording electrooculogram signals, sinusoidal signals of known amplitude and frequency using a signal generator were recorded, following which the electrodes were short circuited. The short circuit was used to check the presence of any offset levels and presence of internal noise sources. Once the integrity of the system was checked, the electrodes were connected to the AMLAB general-purpose biosignal acquisition system.

During recording sessions, the subjects were instructed not to make relative movement of the torso and head, and any other facial movements. This minimized the potential sources of error when determining the angular displacement of the eyes. The electrooculogram was recorded for a number of tests that were designed to assist with the determination of the relationship between electrooculogram and the angular displacement of the eyes. The test procedure detailing each of the tests is described next. Figures 7.5 and 7.6 show an example of the

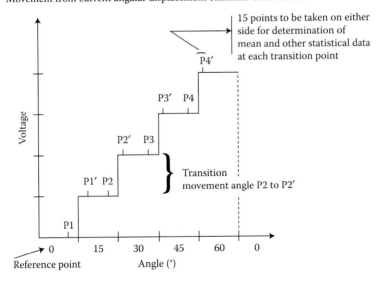

FIGURE 7.5 Schematic description of expected EOG cumulative movement, Type A tests.

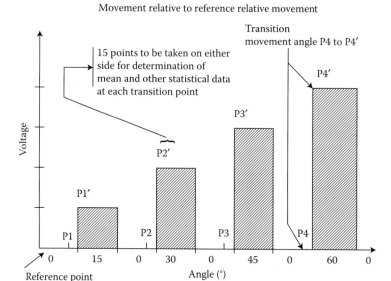

FIGURE 7.6 Schematic description of expected electrooculogram cumulative movement, Type B tests.

electrooculogram for two different conditions: cumulative movement (Type A tests) and relative movement (Type B tests), respectively.

The experimental protocol was standardized for all participants. All recordings commenced and ended with the test subject's eyes fixated on the reference target point, an effective zero. All experiments were repeated three times to obtain sufficient data for the purpose of statistical significance tests. The electrooculogram was also recorded for the eyes fixated on the reference target prior to a change in the direction of the movement, such as during horizontal movement and change in the horizontal direction from left to right. Five seconds of electrooculogram signal was recorded while fixating on the reference target. At other target points, the electrooculogram was recorded for 2 s. Verbal and on-screen cues were given to the subjects.

The tests conducted were designed to

- Determine the relative (peak) and cumulative electrooculogram of the eye during angular displacement in the vertical and horizontal directions
- Determine the characteristics of the electrooculogram as a subject blink, with the eye stationary and moving in the vertical or horizontal directions

- Determine the closeness of the path traced by the eyes compared to the path determined by analysis of the recorded electrooculogram

7.5 Results

Statistical analysis was conducted during this study and the means, medians, and 95% confidence intervals were determined. This enabled the identification of trends in the electrooculogram and the angular error detected. Tables 7.3 and 7.4 tabulate the resolutions for each subject in the horizontal and vertical directions. The results for the 95% confidence intervals show significant variability.

From the results, it is observed that the horizontal direction estimation is significantly more accurate and encouraging,

Table 7.3 Tabulated statistical data, final resolutions, and horizontal electrooculogram movement

Subject	Mean	Standard deviation	Samples	95% Confidence limits	Range of mean Upper limit	Lower limit
A	0.0908	0.0132	45	0.0039	0.095	0.087
B	0.1491	0.0282	36	0.0092	0.158	0.140
C	0.1378	0.0130	42	0.0039	0.142	0.134
D	0.1121	0.0143	46	0.0041	0.116	0.108
E	0.1873	0.0394	41	0.0121	0.199	0.175

Table 7.4 Tabulated statistical data, final resolutions, and vertical EOG movement

Subject	Mean	Standard deviation	Samples	95% Confidence limits	Range of mean Upper limit	Lower limit
A	0.1102	0.0146	30	0.0052	0.115	0.105
B	0.1331	0.0403	30	0.0144	0.148	0.119
C	0.1473	0.0402	30	0.0144	0.162	0.133
D	0.1019	0.0208	29	0.0076	0.110	0.094
E	0.1887	0.0284	30	0.0102	0.199	0.179

although significant intersubject variation is prevalent; two of the subjects have 95% confidence intervals that are greater than those obtained for the other test subjects. In comparison, the vertical direction estimation showed wider variability for all subjects.

The tabulated data demonstrates the potential and limitations of EOG-based eye–gaze detection. However, there are variations when compared with the means and system resolutions (Tables 7.3 and 7.4) that are relatively small for both vertical and horizontal directions.

7.6 Discussion

Analysis of the errors between the expected angular displacement of the eyes, to the angular displacement calculated from the electrooculogram traces recorded for vertical and horizontal movement have revealed a similar trend between the horizontal and vertical directions. The trend, observed in Figures 7.7 and 7.8, has been highlighted by the inclusion of a third-order polynomial. The trend line shows that the errors are tending to increase as the angular displacement approaches the outer test targets, and this angle has been concluded as boarding on the peripheral vision region.

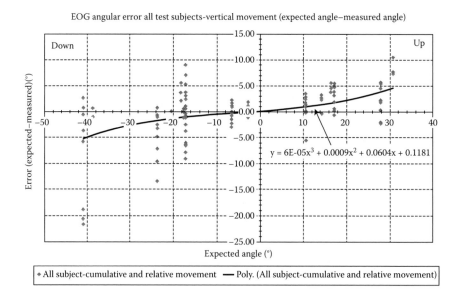

FIGURE 7.7   Vertical, expected electrooculogram angle versus calculated angular error.

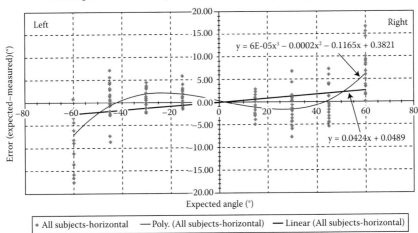

FIGURE 7.8 Horizontal, expected electrooculogram angle versus calculated angular error.

From the results, there also appears to be the existence of a region, where the electrooculogram is approximately linear, while outside this region the relationship appears to be less defined. In the region corresponding to between ±45° for horizontal movement and ±20° for vertical movement, there are less variations.

One cause of errors may be that the distance between the object and the eye was not maintained the same. Independence of distance from a target was assumed for this study, but may in fact need to be investigated. The results of the statistical analysis of the errors are tabulated in Tables 7.5 and 7.6.

Table 7.5 Tabulated statistical data, calculated angular error, and horizontal EOG movement

Subject	Mean (degree)	Standard deviation	Samples	95% Confidence limits	Range of mean Upper limit	Range of mean Lower limit
A	0.9020	2.8347	45.0	0.8282	1.73	0.07
B	−1.2510	5.9811	36.0	1.9538	0.70	−3.20
C	0.0220	3.7196	42.0	1.1249	1.15	−1.10
D	0.4480	3.5284	46.0	1.0196	1.47	−0.57
E	−0.0730	6.9251	41.0	2.1197	2.05	−2.19

Table 7.6 Tabulated statistical data, calculated angular error, and vertical EOG movement

Subjects	Mean (degree)	Standard deviation	Samples	95% Confidence limits	Range of mean	
					Upper limit	Lower limit
A	−0.080	1.7649	30.0	0.632	0.55	−0.71
B	0.450	3.8141	30.0	1.365	1.81	−0.91
C	2.070	2.9766	30.0	1.065	3.14	1.00
D	−3.548	7.8058	29.0	2.841	−0.71	−6.39
E	0.283	2.1967	30.0	0.786	1.07	−0.50

7.7 Limitations of the study

The evidence after the analysis of recorded electrooculogram signals indicates that with appropriate filtering and manipulation, it is possible to obtain a mathematical expression, or data, suitable for input to an HCI. During this study, rapid eye movements between target points were not studied. Rapid movement implies higher frequencies. It is therefore probable that the electrooculogram signals recorded during this study may have contained higher frequencies had the eye movement between target points been faster, this in no way detracts from the validity of conclusions drawn during this study. It is considered that the conclusions, for the slower eye movement, are still applicable for EOG signals that contain higher frequencies.

When the electrooculogram traces were examined, it was concluded that the electrooculogram signal was pseudodeterministic in nature, and as such, the angular displacement at some specific point of time in the future could not be determined. Yet it has been concluded from the evidence obtained during the study that an expression can be derived that will give the expected angle, at the current instant of time. The relationship between EOG voltage and angular displacement of the subject's eyes can only be determined, with confidence, after statistical analysis of a significant number of eye movement tests.

The design of a man–machine interface relies not only on the formulation of a mathematical expression, but also on commands or controls to initiate specific actions. In the simplest case, the interface will trace every eye movement, but this has the disadvantage that it results in small sporadic movements superimposed on the genuine movement. In reality, for many applications, it is only at certain times that movement of an object is required, and that this movement corresponds to the event when the eyes fixate on to a target location.

Analysis of the frequency content using power spectral density (PSD) analysis revealed that it is possible to filter the electrooculogram signals using a narrower band of frequencies than actually used to acquire the electrooculogram signals during this study. The use of a narrower filter band is possible if the maximum velocity of eye movement is considered. The band of frequencies used during this study and the possible narrower band are both at the lower end of the frequency band recommended for use in clinical diagnosis of eye problems. The specific eye movement velocities are of particularly importance if eye blinks are being considered for the initiation of control sequences, as has been proposed by some authors in the literature reviewed.

The results of the current study have shown that a reduction of the filter 3 dB cutoff frequency, from the initial low pass of 5 to 1 Hz, has the potential to reduce analysis errors. The reduction would appear to have its greatest potential in control applications that utilize the differentiated signal or when using neural networks. The lower filter cutoff frequency would assist with denoising of the signal allowing greater recognition of the electrooculogram levels and its features, reducing the complexities of signal analysis and making it easily interpreted by a neural network.

7.8 Discussion: User benefits and limitations

The aforementioned example has shown that EOG has a good relationship with the eye gaze in the horizontal plane. The results also indicate that there is significant variability between subjects and between multiple repetitions. Although this demonstrates the limitations of the system, it also shows the strengths and number of applications. Such a system is easy to deploy, such that an untrained person could connect the user to the EOG device and use it for detecting the gaze of the user. This could be used to control the cursor on the computer screen, or to identify objects in a room, or other diverse range of applications.

The example shows that the system is reasonably reliable and the hardware description shows that it is easy to use and inexpensive. Such a system can be suitable and useful for people who do not have their hands to control the computer or other similar devices, but have the ability to control their gaze.

The example did not include a trigger function, which is essential for the system to obtain a command after identifying the gaze. This, however, may not be difficult, such as the use of eye blink. This would, however, be limited to people who have sufficient control on their eye blink. For those people who are unable to voluntarily blink their eyes, there are also other options such as determining the amount of time for which the user gazes and using a time-based approach.

The other limitation in this system was the need for the user not to move their head. Although this may be acceptable under short-time experimental condition, this would not be acceptable for regular use. There is the need for the system to identify the head movement and subtract this from the eye-gaze angle. Researchers have performed direct subtraction to estimate the location on the screen where the user is gazing. However, such a system has a number of shortcomings because these movements are in three dimensions, making the two-dimensional approximation inaccurate.

There are groups that have attempted to use a lightweight tablet that is fixed to a head-stand and thus the relative angle of the screen location is independent of the head angle. However, such a system suffers from the inflexibility and the weight of the device on the head of the user.

Other methods to overcome this is by the use of a video based on tracking the head of the person using an electromechanical device and identifying relative movement of the eyes by modeling the eye and head of the user. Such a system requires significant calibration and is computationally expensive. However, with the availability of fast computers and the need for user-dedicated devices, this should soon be possible.

One of the shortcomings in these devices has been the movement artifacts. This is often when the contact between the electrodes and the skin is not good, and may happen due to a number of reasons such as (1) the skin was not cleaned prior to electrode applications, (2) electrode adhesiveness gets weak over the time of the experiment, (3) movement, and (4) sweat. To overcome these, it is important that the skin be well cleaned, and the electrodes should be firmly mounted and periodically checked to ensure they are still firmly attached. It is also important that if there are wires, these are firmly secured, and if there is any sweat formation, this is cleaned.

One shortcoming in each of these devices is the user acceptability. While people who are unable to function without such a device would accept it due to lack of choices, and defense personnel may use the device as an integral part of their work; people do find wires hanging from their face disconcerting. Thus, efforts have been made to incorporate the electrodes in devices such as spectacles of the user. Efforts are also being made to have these electrodes be wireless.

References

1. LEIGH RJ, ZEE DS. *The Neurology of Eye Movements*, 2nd Edition. F. A. Davis Company, Philadelphia, 1991.
2. MORGAN SW, PATTERSON J, SIMPSON DG. Utilizing EOG for the measurement of saccadic eye movements. Inaugural Conference of the Victorian Chapter of the IEEE Engineering in Medicine and Biology Society, Victoria, Australia, February 22–23, 1999. Available at: http://www.eng.monash.edu.au/non-cms/ecse/ieee/ieeebio1999/p33.htm. Accessed August 8, 2015.
3. MARMOR MF, BRIGELL MG, WESTALL CA, BACH M. ISCEV standard for clinical electro-oculography (2010 Update). *Documenta Ophthalmologica* 2011:122, 1–7.
4. EVENS WF. *Anatomy and Physiology.* Prentice-Hill, Englewood Cliffs, NJ, 1983.
5. GUYTON AC. *Textbook of Medical Physiology*, 5th Edition. W. B. Saunders Company, Philadelphia, 1976.
6. GIPS J, OLIVIERI, P. EagleEyes: An eye control system for persons with disabilities. Presented at 11th International Conference on Technology and Persons with Disabilities, Los Angeles, California, March 1996. Available at http://www.cs.bc.edu/~gips/EagleEyes1996.pdf. Accessed August 8, 2015.
7. BAREA R, BOQUETE L, MAZO M, LOPEZ E, BERGASA LM. EOG guidance of a wheelchair using neural networks. In *Proceedings of the 15th International Conference on Pattern Recognition,* 2000:4, 668–671.
8. KUNO Y, YAGI T, UCHIKAWA Y. Development of eye pointer with free head-motion. In *Proceedings of the 20th Annual International Conference of the IEEE Engineering in Medicine and Biology Society* 1998:4, 1750–1752.
9. KWON SH, KIM HC. EOG-based glasses-type wireless mouse for the disabled. *Proceedings of the First Joint BMES/EMBS Conference*, Atlanta, GA, October 13–16, 1999.
10. NORRIS G, WILSON E. The Eye Mouse: An eye communication device. In *Proceedings of the IEEE 23rd Northeast Bioengineering Conference*, 1997: 66–67.
11. KAUFMAN AE, BANDOPADHAY A, SHAVIV BD. An eye tracking computer user interface. In *Proceedings IEEE Symposium on Research Frontiers in Virtual Reality* 1993: 120–121.

Further reading

HUGES BA, TAKAHIRA M. ATP-dependent regulation of inwardly rectifying K+ current in bovine retinal pigment epithelial cells. *American Journal of Physiology Society* 1998:275, C1372–C1383.

HUGHES BA, MASAYUKI T, YASUNORI S. An outwardly rectifying K+ current active near the resting potential in human retinal pigment epithelial cells. *American Journal of Physiology* 1995:269, C179–C187.

KUNO Y, YAGI T, UCHIKAWA Y. Biological interaction between man and machine. In *IEEE Conference on Intelligent Robots and Systems, IROS 97* 1997:1, 318–323.

MARMOR MF. From sea lemons to c-wave. *Journal of Cellular Molecular and Neurobiology* 1983:3(4), 285–295.

MARMOR MF. Clinical eletrophysiology of the retinal pigment epithelium. *Documenta Ophthalmologica* 1991:76(4), 301–313.

NIEMEYER G. Selective rod- and cone-ERG responses in retinal degenerations. *Digital Journal of Ophthalmology* 1998:4(10).

RIZZOLO LJ, ZHOU S. The distribution of Na+, K(+)-ATPase and 5A11 antigen in apical microvilli of retinal pigment epithelium is unrelated to alpha-spectrin. *Journal of Cellular Science* 1995:108(Pt 11), 3623–3633.

RIZZOLO I J. Polarization of Na+, K(+)-ATPase in epithelia derived from the neuroepithelium. *International Review of Cytology* 1999:185, 195–235.

STEINBERG RH. Interactions between the retinal pigment epithelium and the neural retina. *Documenta Ophthalmologica* 1985:60(4), 327–346.

CHAPTER EIGHT

Video-based eye tracking

Abstract

It is natural for us humans to direct our gaze to objects of interest and this can lead to a number of technical applications. Machine-based identification of the direction of our gaze has a number of applications suitable for able-bodied and disabled people. People who are unable to effectively use their hands and lack speech can use their eye gaze to control their computers or other associated devices. Thus, the user can move the cursor on the screen, select icons, or even the characters on the keyboard to type and communicate effectively by the machine automatically recognizing the gaze of the person. Although there are various modalities that facilitate machine-based eye-gaze recognition, video-based eye tracking is perhaps the least intrusive. The advantage is that the camera is not located on the face of the individual and may be located at a distance, such as on the computer screen. This technology is significantly matured and there are commercial products available. However, these have limitations such as background and lighting conditions.

8.1 Introduction

Eye detection and tracking is important for many applications such as face recognition, human–computer interface (HCI), and user behavior analysis. The art of automatic machine-based detection of the eye has been perfected, and is routinely done in various airports around the world for identifying travelers based on their biometrics. Eye tracking is where a user's eye movements and the sequence in which the eyes are shifted from one location to another are analyzed. This has clinical and control applications, and researchers are developing new methods to accurately track people's eye movements. The applications range from clinical, social, and behavioral understanding, and for HCI, being very useful for people with reduced motor abilities. The eye-gaze movements can be used to interact and control computerized devices for communication [1].

To track the movement of the eye, there are a number of modalities that have been developed and these can be broadly divided into video-based and bioelectric-based recordings. Each of these has their advantages and limitations and the choice is based on the application. The movement of the eye can be very rapid, in the range of 500 degree/s [2], and although such speeds are not important in some applications, they can be critical in others; tracking the eye at this speed is a challenging task. Other challenges are related to the ambient conditions, location of the sensors, movement of the head, and presence of other people.

Researchers have been investigating techniques to track eye movements using video recording, and various technologies have been developed and implemented in many disciplines as fundamental instruments [3,4]. A general eye detection method follows two steps: (1) locating the face to extract the regions of eye and (2) detecting the eye from the region of interest. Face detection has some constraints such as frontal view, variations in light, and background conditions.

Eye movement is tracked and analyzed to enable an individual to interface with a computer or associated device. Users can position a cursor by looking at the screen and control the movement of the cursor. The selection of the location or the icon can then be made using eye blink or based on the time of gazing. Such interfaces with this capability will be useful for users with feeble muscles or those who lack the ability to control their hands [5].

Video-based eye-gazing analysis systems for HCI are now done in real time and there is software commercially available for this purpose. However, there are a number of unresolved issues such as determining the user's intention, distinguishing between voluntary and involuntary movement, and lighting conditions and background, all of which may lead to inaccurate results. This chapter provides insight to the techniques for tracking eye movements, and an example of the video-based tracking method and its use in HCI applications.

8.2 Background and history

Our eyes are our windows to the world and our major sense organ. They sense the presence of light and convert it into electrical signal, which is then transmitted via the neurons to the brain where it is analyzed to give us the information and perception of the three-dimensional world. The eye has adaptable lens that allows the eye to focus on different depths. The light-sensitive region of the eye is the retina.

Rod and cone cells in the retina allow light perception and vision including various colors. Although the more detailed processing is done by the visual cortex and other areas of the brain, significant analysis takes place in the region of the nerve concentration and where the blood vessels feed the eye, the optic disk, which is often referred to as the blind spot. Our eyes obtain the information of the three-dimensional world on our two-dimensional retina, and thus the direct information obtained by the eye is largely two dimensional. We have two eyes that provide us with stereovision and this facilitates us to get the three-dimensional information. The information of the depth is also superimposed on our vision in our brain based on the spatial model of the environment that is available to us based on other sensors.

The eye converts the optical information to neural information. The brain is attentive to the locations that correspond to the edges, where there is significant change in the color or light intensity. There is also the aspect of movement, where the brain is attentive to the movement of the object in relation to the background. This is perhaps the survival instinct, where we are able to identify movement relative to the background even when our head is in motion.

The eyes are excellent in tracking the movement of other objects. While the eye without any movement is able to identify the movement of objects, when the eye is tracking a moving object, there is movement of the iris cornea and sclera. This is controlled by the muscles of the eye, and gets the sensory information from both, the vision and the ear. The part of the ear senses the movement and position of the body, and sound also identifies the movement of external objects.

There are various methods that have been used to track eye movements since the introduction of eye-tracking technology in 1989 [6]. The following are some of the methods reported in the literature:

- Electrooculogram signal processing techniques, which is based on the differences in electric potential to detect eye movements.

- Historical methods that measure eye movements by fluctuations in an electromagnetic field when the metal coil is moved along with the eyes [7].

- Modern eye-tracking systems use video images of the eye to determine where a person is looking, termed as "point of regard." Many distinguishing features of the eye can be used to infer point of regard, such as corneal reflections (known as Purkinje images), the iris–sclera boundary, and the apparent pupil shape [7].

Eyes can make three different types of motions: (1) horizontal rotation, (2) vertical rotation, and (3) rotation about the visual axis. Most eye movement monitoring techniques only measure the horizontal and vertical rotations, which provide a better output to control a device. These motions can be tracked utilizing the various eye features using image-based tracking methods. These image-based approaches often take advantage of the spectral properties of the eye under near-infrared (NIR) illumination. When NIR light is shone onto the eyes, it is reflected off the different structures in the eye and creates several types of IR illuminated eye features [8,9].

The direct eye localization methods have been classified into three main categories [3]:

1. Shape-based approaches, described by the shape including the iris, contours of pupil, and the exterior shape of the eye.
2. Feature-based shape methods explore the characteristics of the eye to capture a set of distinctive features around the eyes such as the edges, pupil, and cornea reflections.
3. Appearance-based methods detect and track eyes directly using the photometric appearance characterized by the color distribution or filter responses of the eye and its surroundings.

Detection and localization of the eye is now done routinely with number of applications such as biometrics such as for the identity of the person. Eye detection also has applications such as for eye-open condition required for the driver of a vehicle and for detecting when the user of a mobile phone looks at the phone, and the screen gets activated at such a time. Detecting the eye is now routinely done by inbuilt software in laptops, tablets, and mobile phones.

Research has shown that the cognitive or the thought process is related to what a person is looking at and this is termed as eye–mind relationship [10]. In terms of HCI research, this eye–mind process can provide information about a person's attention in relation to a visual display. This can be measured using the different characteristics of the eye movements, such as fixations and decoding the information by tracing eye movements. The process of understanding useful information from eye-movement and eye-tracking methods for HCI involves the following:

- Identifying the "regions of interest" in the display or interface under evaluation, and
- Analyzing the eye movements that fall within the regions of interest areas.

Research has largely focused on the general use of real-time eye movement data in HCI in more conventional user–computer dialogues. Eye movements can also be used in a different way, by itself, or in combination with other input modalities, such as a mouse, keyboard, sensors, or other devices. Eye-tracking research is currently seeking to improve efficiency and enhance the user experience including [11]

- Using eye tracking to control the mouse cursor on wall-sized displays
- Using eye tracking to control a mouse cursor, but also to select items the cursor rests on by focusing on the object
- Controlling digital three-dimensional games by eye gaze
- Gaze interaction in virtual worlds
- Gaze visualizations in three-dimensional environments
- Combining an eye control and speech interface to speed typing

Currently the world's leading vendor of eye tracking and eye control, Tobii has revolutionized eye-tracking technology research in many fields and has enabled communication for thousands of people with special needs. It has developed products such as Tobii Glasses 2 eye tracker (Figure 8.1), which gives researchers the ability to track and record the eye movements to be used for various applications.

This chapter provides an example of an eye-tracking method that can be used as information to control a device for disabled people to communicate. This chapter will also provide an insight into the user requirements and future research on the video-based eye-tracking technology for HCI.

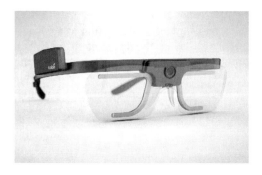

FIGURE 8.1   Tobii Glasses 2 eye tracker. (From Tobii Technology. With permission.)

8.3 An example eye-tracking method

Researchers have demonstrated various video-based eye-tracking techniques in the last decade. They have taken into consideration the lighting conditions, size of the eye, relevant information to be extracted from the image, and other related factors that may affect the accuracy. Some of these factors have been considered in the method explained in the following sections.

8.3.1 Hough transform

The Hough transform was devised by Hough [12]. It is one of the basic methods of identifying the geometry from images in the image processing. Its purpose is to find imperfect objects within a certain class of shapes. The basic principle of Hough transform is that if the curve is given expression in the original image space, the parameter of the curve expression becomes a point in the parameter space. Hence, the detection curve in the original image is transformed into finding the peak value of the voting procedure in parameter space. The original Hough transform was concerned with the identification of a straight line in the image, but later the Hough transform has been extended to identifying arbitrary shapes, circles, and ellipses. This is suitable for an eye-tracking technology.

The following example demonstrates the basic operations of Hough transform better: There is a known line in a black-and-white image (white background and black line), and if we want to calculate the location of the line we can use the equation

$$y = k * x + b$$

where k is the slope constant and b is the intercept.

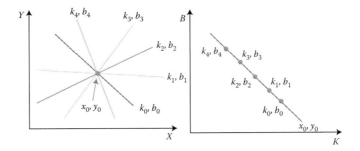

FIGURE 8.2 Point in X–Y plane and in K–B plane.

If given a point $O(x_0, y_0)$ is in the straight line (Figure 8.1), this point will fit in the equation

$$y_0 = k * x_0 + b$$

Now assume that there are many straight lines in the X–Y plane (which represents the original plane in the project) and they all have a common point O, the slope, and intercept of them are k_0, b_0; k_1, b_1; k_2, b_2; k_3, b_3; and k_4, b_4 (details shown in Figure 8.2). Each paired parameter represents a point in the parameter plane, which is called the K–B plane in this case. The five points in the example construct a new straight line in the K–B plane. It is because the five points satisfy the following equation:

$$b = x_0 * k + y_0$$

in the K–B plane. The x_0 becomes the slope and y_0 becomes the intercept parameters of the equation in the K–B plane.

Conceptually, Hough transformation transforms a point in the original image to a line in parameter plane, and transforms a straight line in the original image to a point in parameter plane. In practical application, there is no way to express the linear equation of $x = c$, where the slope of the line is infinite. Hence, the parametric equation

$$p = x * \cos(\theta) + y * \sin(\theta) \text{ replaces}$$

$$y = k * x + b \text{ form}$$

8.3.2 Otsu's method

In computer vision and image processing, Otsu's method is used to automatically perform clustering-based image or the reduction of a gray-level image to a binary image [13]. The algorithm assumes that the image to be the threshold contains two classes of pixels or bimodal histogram in minimal. Then, it uses Equation 8.1 to calculate the threshold to determine the interclass variance

$$g = \omega_f * \omega_b * (\mu_f - \mu_b)^2 \qquad (8.1)$$

where g is the grayscale level that separates the foreground from the background in the image, ω_f is the ratio of target (front part of the image) pixels number over the total pixel number, ω_b indicates the ratio of background pixels over total pixels, μ_f is the average grayscale level for target, and μ_b is the average grayscale level for background.

In this algorithm design, to have higher accuracy in detecting eye during the movement with different backgrounds, Otsu's method provides an improved outcome and is less sensitive to background variations.

8.3.3 Design algorithm

In this algorithm, the first step is to detect the iris. This is based on the observation that the sclera is always brighter than the iris and thus the algorithm detects the edge by a series of points that are located on a circle. This modified algorithm can be described by the following procedure:

1. Resize the image of each frame of video and convert the image into a gradient image.
2. Apply Otsu's method and the Gaussian blur technique to the modified image.
3. Apply the circular Hough transform (CHT) to find the circular shape objects.
4. Identify one maximum area of circle and note the coordinate (x_1, y_1) of the central point of this area (Figure 8.3).
5. Determine the matching second central coordinate (x_2, y_2) point; it must be inside the region of interest
6. If there is no second central coordinate to identify the second eye, return to step 2 and repeat. If the second maximum number has been identified, select this area, then record the coordinate (x_2, y_2) of central point.
7. Compare the radius and the similarity of the two regions using the mean absolute error (MAE) method.
8. If the MAE value is less than the fixed threshold, then the two regions are considered the best match for tracking the eyes. Otherwise return to step 2 and repeat the process.

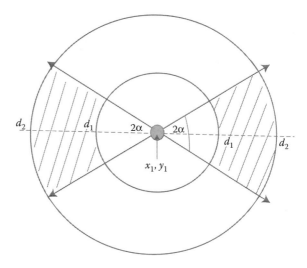

FIGURE 8.3   Region of interest.

The second point (x_2, y_2) can be identified in the shadowed regions shown in Figure 8.3. The following equations present the relation between the first eye and second eye:

$$d_1 \le \sqrt{(x_1 - x_2)^2 + (y_1 - y_2)^2} \le d_2 \tag{8.2}$$

$$\sin \alpha = \frac{|y_1 - y_2|}{\sqrt{(x_1 - x_2)^2 + (y_1 - y_2)^2}}, \quad \alpha \in \left[-\frac{\pi}{6}, \frac{\pi}{6}\right] \tag{8.3}$$

8.3.4 Problems with eye-tracking technique

There are several factors that can influence the accuracy in tracking the eye. Some of these are shown in Figure 8.4 and include

- Varying diameter of iris with different people
- Distance from the camera to the person
- Different lighting backgrounds
- Different shape and size of the eye

To remove those false positives arising due to these factors, measuring the distance of a camera to a person by adding the sensor and computing the expected radius and distance between the two eye sensors may solve this problem. This has been tested with the modified design explained in the next section.

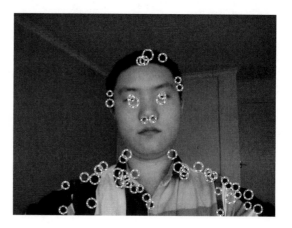

FIGURE 8.4   Resultant images showing the false positives in eye-tracking algorithm.

8.4 Data analysis

8.4.1 Distance detection

Figure 8.5 shows the basic design in detecting the distance. Width marks the dimensions at the distance of a camera to the person. Assuming the angle α is constant, the distance is computed using Equations 8.4 and 8.5.

$$\text{Width} = 2 * \tan \alpha * D \tag{8.4}$$

The iris radius in pixels is

$$R_{\min} = 5 * \left(\frac{\text{Width}_{\text{pixels}}}{\text{Width}} \right), \quad R_{\max} = 7 * \left(\frac{\text{Width}_{\text{pixels}}}{\text{Width}} \right) \tag{8.5}$$

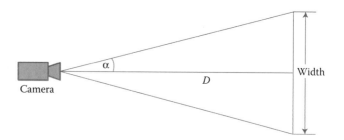

FIGURE 8.5   Plot showing the important variables in calculations.

To test this measure, a simple example of a laser point distance measurement was performed. This technique needs one complementary metal-oxide semiconductor (CMOS) camera and one laser emitter as shown in Figure 8.6. Based on the model shown in Figure 8.5, with fixed height, h, the distance, D, was calculated using the Equation 8.6

$$D = \frac{h}{\tan \theta}, \quad \theta = \text{pfc} * \text{rpc} \tag{8.6}$$

where pfc is the number of pixels from the center to focal plane and rpc is the radians per pixel.

To remove false positives in the eye detection, it is important that the size of the iris and the pupillary distance is accurately measured. This can often be a challenge because different people have different iris sizes. One method to manage the inter-subject differences is the use of circular Hough transform.

Circular Hough transform is an important method to accurately detect the location of the iris. It is based on the common feature that the iris is always darker that the sclera and has a perfect circular shape. Another factor that will affect the eye tracking is the change in the angle of eyes and this angle is due to head movement. The robustness of the method was tested by including the head movement, while tracking the eye. The design of the method to include the head movement is shown in Figure 8.7.

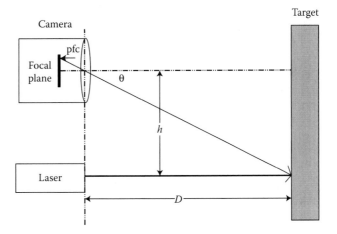

FIGURE 8.6 Distance measurement by using one laser point and one camera.

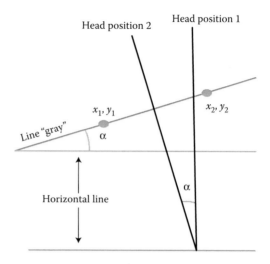

FIGURE 8.7   Angle relations between head and eyes considered in this method. Head position 1 refers to the vertical straight. Head position 2 refers to the head moving left or right, and angle x and y are the coordinates of two eyes' centers.

To track the eye movement by including the factor of head movement was modified based on the geometry of eyes: both iris being the same size and having a similar radius; the fixed pupillary distance; and the angle between two eyes. Although there are other methods that sense the head movement using inertial or electromagnetic sensors, such methods require additional sensors and are intrusive. Further, inertial sensors suffer the shortcomings of temporal drift.

Based on the known anatomy of the head and associated properties, Equations 8.7 and 8.8 have been used in this study

$$d_1 \leq \sqrt{(x_1 - x_2)^2 + (y_1 - y_2)^2} \leq d_2 \tag{8.7}$$

$$\sin \alpha = \frac{|y_1 - y_2|}{\sqrt{(x_1 - x_2)^2 + (y_1 - y_2)^2}}, \quad \alpha \in \left[-\frac{\pi}{6}, \frac{\pi}{6} \right] \tag{8.8}$$

8.5 Results

The results of each step in tracking the eye movement are shown next.

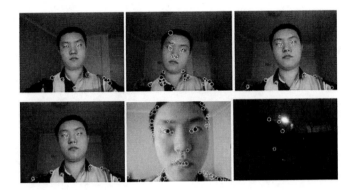

FIGURE 8.8 Image showing results from step 1 to find the circular-shaped objects.

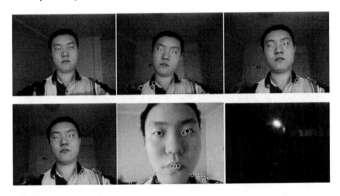

FIGURE 8.9 Image showing results from step 2 by removing some of the false positives.

- Step 1: Apply the circular Hough transform to find the circular-shaped objects. Results from this step are shown in Figure 8.8.
- Step 2: Remove the false positives by identifying the possible locations of the eye. The results from this step are shown in Figure 8.9.
- Step 3: Compare the radius of the remaining coordinates and applying MAE to measure similarity. The results are shown in Figure 8.10, where the eye was tracked accurately even though the head moved right or left at an angle.

8.6 Discussion: User benefits and limitations

Eye tracking has been used to evaluate the user behavior and the interface usability in many HCI-based research and

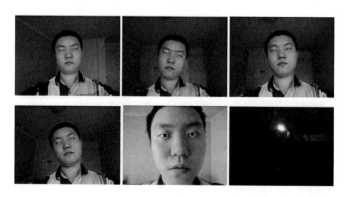

FIGURE 8.10 Image showing results from step 3 by applying MAE to measure similarity, which includes the head movement.

applications. In the HCI applications, it has been predominantly used as a direct control interface for communication applications. Eye-tracking research is currently leading toward developing devices for people with disabilities where they can communicate through their eyes. However, there other applications where eye tracking is routinely used, such as for virtual reality environments, computer games, and defense. More recent applications include the use of eye tracking for psychological experiments, marketing, and social experiments.

Eye tracking is now a matured technology and there are a number of commercial devices and systems. One driving force is the availability of inexpensive good digital cameras, which are often embedded inside laptop computers, tablets, and mobile phones. Although there are several companies that are marketing these devices, Tobii is an example of one leading company that has been researching and developing eye-tracking technology; SenoMotoric Instruments is an example of a new company with some novel applications. These companies have developed various products to analyze human behavior and their usability of devices, for example, the Tobii eye tracker (Figure 8.1). Tobii has developed and marketed products to conduct research in real-world environments in fields ranging from psychology, infant, and reading research to neuroscience and vision research. Eye movements are often used in HCI studies involving people with disabilities who can use only their eyes for input. Tobii eye control technology has already revolutionized the lives of thousands of people with disabilities [11]. Some of their tracking technology is shown in Figure 8.11.

Researchers [14] have used eye-gaze-based interaction to help autistic children learn social skills when they maintain

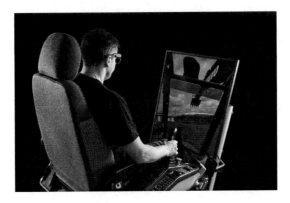

FIGURE 8.11   Tobii eye track technology simulator. (From Tobii Technology. With permission.)

eye contact while communicating. Hornof et al. [15] designed a software called "EyeDraw" to enable children with severe motor impairments to draw with their eyes. Their study demonstrated and reported that it requires detailed analysis and understanding of fundamental human-perceptual constraints and oculomotor control to create HCIs for new eye control of software applications.

Eye trackers are sensitive to the instrumentation and thus the software and hardware are often not stand-alone, which can limit the usage. There are also the shortcomings such as the effect of eyewear (e.g., hard contact lenses, bifocal and trifocal glasses, and glasses with supercondensed lenses) and some eye makeup of the participants that can interrupt the normal path of a reflection. There may also be problems tracking people with very large pupils or "lazy eye," such that their eyelid obscures part of the pupil and makes it difficult to identify. Calibration is required to maintain the accurate point of measurement due to the differences in eye movements between participants on identical tasks. Visual distractions (e.g., colorful or moving objects around the screen or in the testing environment) should also be eliminated, as these will inevitably contaminate the eye-movement data [16]. Based on the literature, future developments in eye tracking should concentrate on accurate tracking, making users feel more comfortable, and cost-effectiveness for consumers.

Another limitation of video-based eye tracking is for people who may suffer from nystagmus. Such people suffer rapid and involuntary eye movement, which may occur regularly or be very occasional. Although people who suffer regular nystagmus are unable to use the device, the difficulty is associated with those people who have the condition under some specific conditions and in such cases there can be erroneous outcomes. There is the need for identifying such conditions to ensure that the system does not identify an incorrect command. People have attempted to use temporal filtering methods to ensure that such events are filtered.

References

1. Visual Perception Laboratory. Eye movements. Available at: http://www.cis.rit.edu/vpl/eye_movements.html. Accessed December 15, 2014.
2. POOLE A, BALL LJ. Eye tracking in human-computer interaction and usability research: Current status and future prospects. In *Encyclopedia of Human Computer Interaction*, edited by C Ghaoui, 211–219. Idea Group, Pennsylvania, 2005.
3. BALYA D, ROSKA T. Face and eye detection by CNN algorithms. *Journal of VLSI Signal Processing* 1999:23, 497–511.
4. SMITH P, SHAH M, DA VITORIA LOBO N. Determining driver visual attention with one camera. *IEEE Transactions on Intelligent Transportation Systems* 2003:4(4), 205–218.
5. JACOB RJK, KARN KS. Eye tracking in human-computer interaction and usability research: Ready to deliver the promises. In *The Mind's Eye: Cognitive and Applied Aspects of Eye Movement Research*, edited by J Hyön, R Radach, and H Deubel, 573–605. Elsevier, Amsterdam, 2003.
6. RAYNER K, POLLATSEK A. *The Psychology of Reading.* Prentice Hall, Engle-Wood Cliffs, NJ, 1989.
7. DUCHOWSKI AT. *Eye Tracking Methodology: Theory and Practice.* Springer-Verlag Ltd., London, 2003.
8. CHERABIT N, CHELALI FZ, DJERADI A. Circular Hough transform for iris localization. *Science and Technology* 2012:2(5), 114–121.
9. CHAKRABARTI A, HIRAKAWA K, ZICKLER T. Color constancy beyond bags of pixels. In *IEEE Conference on Computer Vision and Pattern Recognition* 2008: 1–6.
10. JUST MA, CARPENTER PA. Eye fixations and cognitive processes. *Cognitive Psychology* 1976:8, 441–480.
11. Tobii. Human–computer interaction and eye tracking. Available at: http://www.tobii.com/eye-tracking-research/global/research/human-computer-interaction/. Accessed June 17, 2015.
12. HOUGH PVC. Machine analysis of bubble chamber pictures. In *Proceedings of International Conference on High Energy Accelerators and Instrumentation* 1959: 554–558.
13. OTSU N. A threshold selection method from gray-level histograms. *IEEE Transactions on Systems, Man, and Cybernetics* 1979:9(1), 62–66.

14. RAMLOLL R, TREPAGNIER C, SEBRECHTS M, FINKELMEYER A. A gaze contingent environment for fostering social attention in autistic children. In *Proceedings of the Eye Tracking Research and Applications Symposium*, 19–26. ACM, New York, 2004.

15. HORNOF AJ, CAVENDER A, HOSELTON R. EyeDraw: A system for drawing pictures with eye movements. In Proceedings of ASSETS 2004: *The Sixth International ACM SIGACCESS Conference on Computers and Accessibility*, 86–93. ACM Press, New York, 2004.

16. GOLDBERG HJ, WICHANSKY AM. Eye tracking in usability evaluation: A practitioner's guide. In *The Mind's Eye: Cognitive and Applied Aspects of Eye Movement Research*, edited by J Hyönä, R Radachand, H Deubel H, 493–516. Elsevier, Amsterdam, 2003.

CHAPTER NINE

Speech for controlling computers

Abstract

Voice recognition technologies for computer and machine control applications are growing due to the flexibility of speech-based communication. There are a number of devices and software commercially available and used for commanding computers, lights in a building, and toys, to name a few. This chapter discusses some of these technologies in the context of aids for people with disabilities, and identifies the associated applications and limitations.

9.1 Introduction

Speech facilitates human beings to communicate effectively with others. The complexity of human speech makes it possible to communicate complex ideas and is often considered as the defining strength of humans over animals. Use of speech to interact with machines is a much desired option because this will facilitate the user with the ability to command it for complex functions. For effective speech-based computer interaction, the computer has to understand the desired commands. Some of the methods that are used for speech analysis are simple in design and operation, while others are state of the art and computationally complex.

Speech is rich and complex, and it is dependent on number of factors. Some of these are intrinsic to the speaker such as what is being spoken, who is the speaker, and how is the speaker speaking. Then there is the effect of background conditions, room acoustics, and the hardware properties of the microphone. The listener is often able to simultaneously obtain all of this information and identify who is the speaker, what is being spoken, the emotional state of the speaker, and the acoustics in the region. Thus, the desired speech-based computer interaction should be suitable for all of these functions.

The accuracy of any conversation is dependent on factors such as the presence of background noise, other speakers in the vicinity, and acoustics. People are able to understand what is being spoken even when these conditions are not suitable by observing facial and lip movement, and knowing the context of the conversation. However, factors such as lack of knowledge of the context, different accents, and altered speed of the speech can make it difficult for people to understand what was spoken.

Speech is complex, and with the added factors such as room acoustics and noise, speech-based interactions always have a level of uncertainty and this is also the case in computer-based interaction. There are inherent possibilities of error and this is enhanced when message is complex. Computer-based speech command recognition is not trivial and there are several sophisticated algorithms and techniques that have been developed over the past decades. Some of these techniques are discussed in this chapter.

9.2 History of speech-based machine commands

One of the simplest speech-based machine controls is based on the presence of sound above a threshold. Such a system will use the intensity of the audio signal to perform a simple function. The user needs to make a sound above a certain intensity, and this will trigger the machine to perform an action. Although such systems were simple to implement, they were typically only suitable for extremely trivial situations, and very sensitive to the presence of background and other artifact sounds. Enhancement of such a system is the use of filters that reduce the background noise, and filters in sounds that have spectral properties similar to the human voice. However, changing conditions would alter the noise properties and the reliability of such systems can be poor because these may trigger machine command due to background noise.

To overcome the changing conditions, adaptive filters have been introduced. Such techniques reduce the background noise even when the conditions such as room acoustics or the presence of different sources of noise are introduced. Such improvements allow the simple threshold-based systems with a small vocabulary of machine commands, and can be trained and tailored for the individual user. These are suitable for performing some machine commands. However, these were unsuitable for performing complex tasks such as speech-to-text conversion and dictating to a computer.

Speech-based machine control systems that are suitable for performing complex tasks require machine-based speech recognition. This is often referred to in the literature as "automatic speech recognition" (ASR). This has number of applications for people with special needs, and it is also widely used for applications such as "speech to text," often used for transcribing.

ASR systems may be speaker independent or trained for an individual. The speaker-dependent ASR requires speaker voice samples to train the system, whereas the speaker-independent ASR does not require this training. Typically, the ones that require speaker training require the speaker to speak a small set of words, and the system uses this to model other speech characteristics, fine-tuning the algorithms, and these features are saved for further use. More often, the speaker-trained systems are more accurate compared with the speaker-independent ASR.

Many recent ASR systems developed for transcribing are capable of handling complex vocabulary and can work within a defined context, though some are based on the individual characters in a language. Research has shown that most speakers use only a small vocabulary and recent advancements have developed the system to tailor the vocabulary to the individual speaker, thereby reducing the error.

9.3 Automatic speech recognition (ASR)

Machine-based speech command recognition requires three steps: noise removal, speech feature extraction, and classification. To better understand these methods for machine-based speech command recognition, understanding the speech production is important. This is described in the following sections.

9.3.1 Digitization of sound signal The first step in computer-based speech command recognition requires the digitization of the sound signal that is recorded by the microphone. To ensure accurate identification of the speech, it is important that the digitization step is accurate and does not introduce any noise. There are number of factors that have to be considered such as sampling rate and sample bit resolution.

The sampling rate, in most cases, can be based on Nyquist criterion, where the signal is sampled at more than twice the maximum frequency of interest. In most cases, the relevant speech signal is in the range of 50–5000 Hz, and thus a sampling rate of around 10,000 is sufficient. However, many signal-recording systems have their own sampling rates, in the range of 4000–43,100. When digitizing the signal, it is important to note that signal spectrum often has a long tail, far beyond half the sampling rate. This is referred to as aliasing and results in noise. As is shown later, anti-aliasing filters are required to filter this prior to sampling the signal.

The bit-resolution is based on number of factors, but the quality of the microphone is perhaps the most important. Most computers allow for the bit-sample of around 24 bits, or resolution of nanoparts of the signal, 8 or 16 bits are in general sufficient for most applications, with resolutions in milli- or microparts of the signal.

9.4   Speech denoising methods

All speech-recording devices are susceptible to noise. Noise may be due to single source, or a number of sources, and may have a range of distributions and properties. It can be random or white noise with no coherence, or coherent noise introduced by the hardware or processing software. It also may be due to inherent properties of the acoustic properties of the recording environment.

Suppressing unwanted sounds, such as background sounds or other artifacts to obtain pure speech signal, is an essential step prior to obtaining speech features. There are several methods for filtering the signal to obtain the speech while reducing the background noise. One of the simplest methods is based on spectral filtering, where the noise is considered to be stationary. However, in many real conditions, the noise is not stationary, and more recent techniques are adaptive filtering based. One difficulty with the spectral-based methods is the assumption that speech has different a spectrum compared with background noise, and this is often not correct, such as when the background noise is due to other human speech. Recent advancements have resulted in the use of entropy or information-based filtering methods that allow the separation of speech of different speakers. A brief description of these noise suppression techniques is mentioned in the next sections.

9.4.1 Spectral-based filtering

Random white noise would have a spectrum ranges from low to high frequency, and with overlap of the speech signal. One technique to suppress the noise is to filter the recording that is outside the main spectral region of interest, which is often considered to be between 50 and 5000 Hz. Other noises that may corrupt the signal can be narrow band noise generated by the presence of monotonic sounds created by motors in the vicinity or nonlinear properties of the circuit components.

Spectral filters may be interpreted in the time domain or frequency domain. In the frequency domain, there is multiplication of the spectrum of the signal with that of the filter, whereas in the time domain, this may be interpreted as the convolution of the impulse response with the signal. When selecting the suitable filter, there are a number of factors that have to be considered.

Types of filters include low pass, high pass, band pass, and notch. There are also differences related to the order, which determines the sharpness in the cutoff between the accepted and rejected frequencies. Other factors that influence the selection of filters are the presence of ripples in either the stopband or the passband of the filter, phase shift, and delays in the filters.

Spectral filters can be in hardware or software, referred to as the digital filters. With greatly enhanced computational properties, digital filters are routinely used, though there are many situations where the electronic circuit-based filters are essential. One such application where the filter has to be hardware-based is the anti-aliasing filters.

9.4.2 Noise profile

As a first step of denoising the audio recording, a portion of the recording that does not have any speech is selected and the spectrum of this is observed. This indicates the background noise spectrum. The next step is to observe the spectrum of the speech signal and compare the two signals; the spectrum that can be removed for effective noise reduction has to be identified. Often, this will require compromise where in the first step, we select a portion of our sound that contains all noise and no signal; in other words, select the part that is silent except for the noise. Taking the spectrum of this identifies the type of filter that is required to eliminate or reduce the noise.

9.4.3 Low-pass filter

A low-pass filter (LPF) passes that part of the signal with frequency lower than a certain cutoff frequency while stopping or attenuating signals with higher frequencies. Thus, the output of the LPF contains the trends of the signals, while some of the sharpness is removed. They provide a smoother form of a signal, removing the short-term fluctuations, leaving the longer-term trend. LPFs are referred to as treble cut filters and are used for removing high-frequency noise. It is essential that they be added before any signal is sampled to prevent any anti-aliasing noise.

LPFs are in general considered in frequency domain, with the shape and parameters of the spectrum defining the filter. However, it can be considered in time domain. While in frequency domain, the spectrum of the filter is multiplied with that of the signal to obtain the output; in time domain, this requires the convolution of the signal with the impulse response. The hardware implementation of these filters is generally a combination of resistances and capacitances, while the software implementation may also be considered to be an averaging operation.

The shape of the spectrum of the filter defines the properties. One important factor is the sharpness of the shape of the spectrum, which indicates the change and the rate of attenuation, as a function of frequency depends on the filter design, often based on the order of the filter. In time domain, the impulse response of the LPF integral is zero.

9.4.4 Anti-aliasing filter

Prior to digitizing the signal, it is important to ensure that the signal does not have any frequency content that is greater than half the sampling rate. The presence of any such "tail" of the spectrum results in noise being added to the signal. For this purpose, an analog LPF circuit has to be placed before the signal is sampled. This is referred to as the anti-aliasing filters.

9.4.5 High-pass filter

A filter that removes the low-frequency content of the signal and passing the high-frequency content is termed as the high-pass filter (HPF). These filters are also called a high-cut filter or treble cut filter. These filters have the spectrum that is the mirror image of the LPF. These filters keep the sharpness while removing the trends of the signal and may also be considered the bass-removal filters.

In the hardware setting, in the simplest form, HPFs may be considered as a capacitor in series of the signal, and are required to remove the direct current (DC) bias that may exist in some devices such as the microphones. In the software, these may be considered as the "difference" filters. The shape of the filter spectrum is dependent on factors such as the order of the filter.

9.4.6 Band-pass filter

Most real applications require the selection of the signal where the very low and the very high frequencies of the signal are removed. The very low frequencies correspond to factors such as DC drift caused by capacitance or bias voltages, while high frequency signals correspond to noise due to the circuits or the environment. Thus, an appropriate combination of the LPF and HPF result in the band-pass filters, which is often used for many audio applications.

9.4.7 Notch filter In some situations, the noise can have narrow band spectrum, which is located in the middle of the signal spectrum. This may happen for a number of reasons such as resonance in a circuit, leading to a noisy monotone riding on top of the recording. Other causes of narrow band noise may also be the presence of some musical instrument or a machine in the background. Removing this requires a narrow band notch filter that allows all frequencies to pass without attenuation except the narrow band. Often, notch filters may be in series with band-pass filters to remove the low- and high-frequency noise and the narrow-band noise located in the middle of the band-pass spectrum.

9.4.8 Mean and median filter Mean filters can be considered similar to LPFs. They are used to remove impulsive noise. However, whereas standard global filtering techniques like low-pass filtering do not differentiate between impulse corrupted samples and uncorrupted samples, mean and median filters operate on a localized area and smooth the impulsive samples. Median filters have the advantage that they are not affected by large impulses that may affect the mean filters. However, implementation of mean filters is simpler compared with the median filters.

9.4.9 Adaptive filter The use of filters mentioned earlier is based on the assumptions of signal and noise properties being stationary. It is assumed that the spectrum of the noise and the signals remain unchanged over time. However, in most real-world situations, this is not accurate and the spectral properties may change significantly. To ensure that the noise is effectively removed from the recordings, adaptive filters are used.

Adaptive filters have the ability to adapt to the conditions. These may be dynamic and continuously adapt over time to changing conditions, or may adapt at the start of a situation. These are generally digital filters and may have linear or nonlinear transfer function with the properties that are dynamically controlled. The transfer function is controlled by variable parameters to adjust the spectrum of the filter based on a selected optimization algorithm. Adaptive filters are closed-loop systems that use feedback to refine the transfer function.

The effectiveness of these filters is based on the choice of the feedback or error parameters, and is often referred to as the cost function of the filter. The optimization algorithm reduces the overall error based on the choice of the cost functions.

9.4.10 Kalman filter

The Kalman filter was developed and enhanced by Kalman [1], Thiele [2], and Swerling [3]. It tracks the estimated state of the system, and manages the system model with multiple output parameters using linear quadratic estimation (LQE) to optimize the system. These readings are a series of measurements observed over time, containing random noise and other inaccuracies, and produce estimates of unknown variables that tend to be more precise than those based on a single measurement alone. The Kalman filter operates recursively on streams of noisy input data to produce a statistically optimal estimate of the underlying system state.

The Kalman filter algorithm is a two-step process: prediction and update. The prediction step estimates the current state variables, along with their uncertainties. The outcome of the next measurement, corrupted with noise, is used to update the system to minimize the error using a weighted average, biased to estimates with higher certainty. The algorithm is recursive and can run in real time, updating the system over time. These techniques are suitable for biometric applications to identify the speaker.

9.5 Speech analysis fundamentals

Human process audio signal and recognize the speech, emotions, and identity of the speaker. Human hearing consists of the ear, cochlea, and a complex set of neural pathways that identify the foreground activity from the background activity and the direction of the speaker. We understand the message in the speech even when there is noise or multiple speakers. We also have the ability to put the speech in context of the environmental conditions, and all this is performed in real time. However, machine-based analysis of the speech to determine the command of the speaker is not trivial and requires multiple steps. After the first step of cleaning the signal by removing the noise from the speech signal, the cleaned signal is analyzed to obtain suitable features that best represent the signal. These features are specific to the applications, and hence it is important to select the most appropriate feature set for the application. These features have to be classified by the computer to identify or interpret the spoken command. Determining the suitable feature set and classification method is important for successful recognition of the speech command.

Over the past five decades, numerous features for speech analysis have been proposed. While the commonality of all features is the frequency content of the signal, there have been significant improvements over the past few decades. Though some of the earliest methods included the use of correlation in time domain, such techniques were largely discontinued due to significant time-based differences. One common factor that is recognized in speech analysis is that the spectrum of the signal changes over the duration of the speech, and its envelope, presence of harmonics, and temporal changes are the parameters that have to be analyzed.

Some of the earlier attempts used the time and spectrum envelope of the signal; the sensitivity of such systems was very poor, and they were effective only in a noise-free environment with limited vocabulary and with the speaker being expected to speak at a specific speed. Some of the improvements were targeting normalization of the temporal and spectral envelopes to make the systems robust to changes to factors such as speed of speaking and differences among people. There have also been significant improvements in the use of classifiers that incorporate the contextual information.

Studies have incorporated the knowledge of how humans produce speech and how we hear. To obtain the suitable features and classification techniques, it is important to understand how people speak and hear. For this purpose, speech production and hearing models have been developed. One such model for speech production is called the source-filter model, and one model for hearing is the place hearing model. To obtain appropriate classification techniques, speech has been considered in terms of substructures, the phonemes. Each of these techniques with the different signal features and classification are described in the following sections.

9.6 Subsections of speech: Phonemes

A phoneme is a basic unit that describes the sound with the fundamental component of a language. The study of phoneme describes the organization of speech sound in context of a language to form meaningful units of the language, which, in general are the words. In general, changes in the phonemes cause a change in the words being described, and words where there is only one different phoneme are referred to as the minimal pair.

Some languages are called phonetic where the phonemes closely relate to the spellings, and the example of such a language is Sanskrit. English is not known to be a phonetically precise language, and in such languages, there is no specific and direct relationship between the written word structure and the spoken word. In such cases, the phoneme has to be considered in context such as the utterances before or after that phoneme to develop the word. Thus, there is need for memory and forward mapping for machine-based speech sounds interpretation.

Over the past few decades, a set of tools have been developed that provide the mapping and interaction of different phonemes and for the purpose of computer interaction such as machine-based speech-to-text generator and transcribing. Although some of these are generic, they are often language specific. Phonemes have been described in number of subgroups, but these can be largely described in two classes: vowels and consonants. These are described next.

9.6.1 Vowels

Vowels are the sounds made by free passage of breath through the larynx and the oral cavity. When vowel sound is being produced, the shape of the mouth does not change, and the signal can be considered stationary, where the spectral properties remain the same during the duration.

Different vowels are distinguished by formants, which is the spectral peaks of the sound spectrum of the voice. Formant also indicates an acoustic resonance of the human vocal tract and thus it is useful for modeling the vocal track of an individual and for applications such as biometrics. It is often measured as an amplitude peak in the frequency spectrum of the sound, using a spectrogram. Formants are gender and age dependent, with females and children typically having higher formants.

9.6.2 Consonants

During the production of the consonants, the breath is partly obstructed by the oral cavity and there may be movement of the mouth. The sound is produced by constriction and the signal does not have stationary properties.

9.7 How people speak: Speech production model

Human speech is produced when air is forced through the larynx, mouth, and nostrils by the lungs. The lungs can be considered as the power generator, the larynx produces the fundamental frequencies, and the shape of the mouth and lips can be considered as the filters that generate the complex frequency structure of the sound. Such a view of speaking is referred to as the source-filter model. Such a model sees speech production as a combination of three separate sections: sound power or lungs; sound source such as the vocal cords; and acoustic filter, which is the vocal tract. Such a model has been found to be very useful in a number of applications because of its relative simplicity while being significantly detailed. The basic model is shown in Figure 9.1. The source-filter model is used in both speech synthesis and speech analysis.

There are two types of speech: the voiced and the unvoiced. The voiced speech is produced when the vocal cords tense together and vibrate as the air expels through the glottis due to pressure. The frequency spectrum contains the fundamental frequency f_0 (pitch) and harmonics, with spectrum decays at a rate of approximately −12 dB/octave. An adult male pitch is in the range of 50–250 Hz (average 120 Hz), and an adult female's average pitch is about 225 Hz. Children's pitch is higher and the average pitch is 265 Hz.

The implementation of the source-filter model of speech production models the sound source as a periodic impulse train for voiced speech, or white noise for unvoiced speech. The vocal tract filter is, in the simplest case, approximated by an all-pole filter, where the coefficients are obtained by performing linear prediction to minimize the mean-squared error in the speech signal to be reproduced. Convolution of the excitation signal with the filter response produces the synthesized speech.

The unvoiced speech is produced by a turbulent airflow through the constriction of the vocal tract (unvoiced excitation). In the production of the unvoiced speech, the vocal folds do

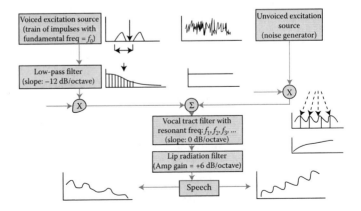

FIGURE 9.1 Basic model of speech production.

not vibrate. This turbulent airflow produces acoustic noise that is essentially white and can therefore be considered as having a flat continuous spectrum. Different phonemes can be distinguished by spectral shape and properties of the formants. Vowels have at periodic glottal excitation, approximated by a set of harmonics in the frequency domain and an impulse train in the time domain, and a fixed filter characteristic based on tongue position and lip protrusion. Some consonants such as fricatives are produced by the unvoiced excitations.

The sound modifiers for the voiced and unvoiced speech are the vocal tract cavities (the oral cavity and the nasal cavity), lips, jaw, tongue, and velum. Movement of those elements changes the shape of the vocal tract, which leads to changes of its acoustic properties, namely, the resonant frequencies called formants. The vocal tract works as a time-varying band-pass filter with constant amplitudes for each frequency band.

The lips radiation works effectively as a HPF with a steady spectrum and amplitudes increasing at about +6 dB/octave across frequencies. The average spectrum of the voiced speech shows decay of amplitude with frequency at an average −6 dB/octave. The overall average spectrum of the unvoiced speech shows an increase of amplitude with frequency at an average ratio of +6 dB/octave.

9.8 Place principle hearing model

The cochlea can be considered as the transducer in the ear, where the sound waves are converted into the neural signals in the form of electrical impulses. These are conducted through the auditory nerve to the auditory region of the brain. Pressure waves enter the cochlea at the oval window travel through the scala vestibuli along Reissner's membrane and through the narrow gap at the apex to continue through the scala tympani along the basilar membrane to the round window where the pressure is released. The basilar membrane has a large number of tiny hair cells to which auditory nerve endings are attached. The mechanical vibrations of the basilar membrane stimulate the hair cells, which transform them into trains of electrical impulses conducted through the auditory nerve to the brain.

The basilar membrane has location-specific spectral properties and performs spectral analysis of the incoming signal. The spectrum of the speech signal is coded on the neural signals

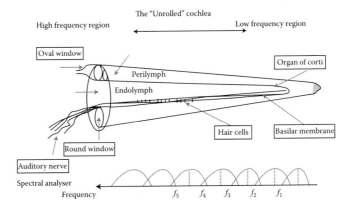

FIGURE 9.2 Model showing peak of the vibration occurs at different places along the basilar membrane for different frequencies.

in the audio nerves. The peak of the vibration occurs at different places along the basilar membrane for different frequencies (see Figure 9.2). The base of the membrane is tuned to low frequencies and the apex responds to high frequencies.

The perception of hearing is not a direct function of the strength of the vibration, but the relationship is complex and dependent on the frequency of the sound. The relationship of the human hearing threshold is a function of frequencies, and the lowest threshold is in the range of 1000–3000 Hz. Thus, the frequencies that are important for human hearing can be identified, and this relationship between frequencies of sound with perception has been described by logarithmic function.

9.9 Features selection for speech analysis

Speech sound needs to be appropriately represented by suitable features. There are factors of sound that are relevant such as the spectrum, the presence of formants, and the temporal changes of the spectrum. There is also the need for appropriate segmentation of the signal to identify the start and the end of the speech sound. Some of the features that are currently used for speech analysis are linear predictive analysis (LPC), linear predictive cepstral coefficients (LPCC), perceptual linear predictive (PLP) coefficients, Mel-frequency cepstral coefficients (MFCC), power spectral analysis (FFT), mel scale cepstral analysis (MEL), and its variants. Some of these are discussed in the following sections.

9.9.1 Power spectral analysis

The power spectrum of the speech signal is one of the common features used for speech signal analysis. This describes the frequency content of the signal as it changes over time. The first step toward computing the power spectrum of the speech signal is to perform a discrete Fourier transform (DFT). A DFT computes the frequency information of the equivalent time domain signal. Since a speech signal contains only real point values, we can use a real-point fast Fourier transform (FFT) for increased efficiency. The resulting output contains both the magnitude and phase information of the original signal. Although this is a useful feature of speech, it often gets distorted because of the presence of high frequency components obtained due to high sampling rates such as 44.1 kHz. To overcome this, the logarithm of the spectrum has been used to model loudness perception.

9.9.2 Linear predictive coding (LPC)

LPC is considered as a powerful speech analysis technique and it is also useful for encoding quality speech at a low bit rate. The underpinning theory is that the speech production can be modeled and the linear combination of the past speech samples can be the basis for approximating future samples.

Linear prediction is based on the model of human speech production and uses a conventional source-filter speech production model where the glottal, vocal tract, and lip radiation transfer functions are integrated into one all-pole filter to simulate the acoustics of the vocal tract. Using the approach of minimizing the sum of the squared differences between the original speech signal and the estimated speech signal over a finite duration, LPC is generated. This could be used to give a unique set of predictor coefficients. These predictor coefficients are estimated in every frame, which is normally 20 ms long.

The LPC analysis of each frame involves the decision-making process of voiced or unvoiced. The pitch is detected using a range of algorithms to obtain the correct periodicity and pitch frequency. The resultant vector is the input to the classifier.

9.9.3 Cepstral analysis

Speech is composed of an excitation source and vocal tract system components. There are multiple parameters such as what is being spoken and the model of who is speaking it. To determine what is being spoken, it is essential that excitation and vocal track properties be separated. Cepstral analysis identifies parameters to separate the speech into its source and system components without any *a priori* knowledge about the source and the system.

According to the source filter theory of speech production, there are two components of speech: voiced and unvoiced. The voiced sounds are produced by exciting the time varying system characteristics with a periodic impulse sequence and unvoiced sounds are produced by exciting the time varying system with a random noise sequence. The resulting speech can be considered as the convolution of the respective excitation sequence and vocal tract filter characteristics. If $e(n)$ is the excitation sequence and $h(n)$ is the impulse response of the vocal tract filter, then the speech sequence $s(n)$ is a result of the convolution in the time domain or multiplication in the frequency domain.

Multiplication of the spectrum of the excitation and system filter characteristics expressed in the frequency domain is the same as the convolution of the time series and the impulse response in the time domain. To perform speech analysis of this sequence, $s(n)$ has to be deconvolved to obtain the excitation and vocal tract components, which may also be performed in the frequency domain using multiplication and thus not requiring integration. For this purpose, multiplication of the two components in the frequency domain has to be converted to a linear combination of the two components.

The word *cepstral* is nearly the word *spectral* written front to back. Cepstral analysis is used for transforming the multiplied source and system components in the frequency domain to the linear combination of the two components in the cepstral domain. The spectrum of the signal is first represented on the log scale and the spectrum of this is obtained. This highlights the formants of the signal and represents the signal source properties.

9.9.4 Basic principle

The flow chart in Figure 9.3 shows the steps that are required to obtain the cepstral representation of any given short-term speech signal. $s(n)$ is the voiced frame considered and $x(n)$ is the windowed frame obtained by a hamming window. $|x(\omega)|$ is the spectrum of the windowed signal $x(n)$. Taking the log of the spectrum, $\log|x(\omega)|$ represents the log magnitude of the spectrum. The cepstrum, $c(n)$ is obtained by taking the inverse discrete Fourier transform (IDFT) and this contains vocal tract components. The domain of $c(n)$ is referred to as

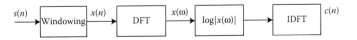

FIGURE 9.3 Block diagram representing computation of cepstrum.

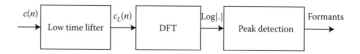

FIGURE 9.4   Block diagram representing low-time liftering.

quefrency and even though the variable, n, is used, this is not in the time domain. As the cepstrum is derived from the log magnitude of the linear spectrum, it is symmetrical in the quefrency domain.

The cepstrum is analyzed using the liftering operation, which is similar to the filtering operation in the frequency domain. Liftering selects a desired quefrency region for analysis by multiplying the cepstrum by a rectangular window at the desired position of the quefrency. Similar to the frequency domain, there are two types of liftering: low-time liftering and high-time liftering. The low-time liftering operation extracts the vocal tract characteristics, and high-time liftering is performed to get the excitation characteristics.

The important vocal tract parameters like formant location and bandwidth can be computed from the vocal-tract spectrum. The formant locations can be estimated by picking the peaks from the smooth vocal tract spectrum. The block diagram given in Figure 9.3 shows the process of formant estimation using low-time liftering. Figure 9.4 shows the computation of low-time liftering.

9.10   Speech feature classification

The features of the speech signal have to be classified by the machine to identify the spoken word or command. There are number of options, and the selection of these is dependent on the applications. The use of statistical methods may be suitable for simple applications such as for identifying the presence or absence of speech, and may be useful for triggering applications such as switching on the lights in a room, but such techniques are not suitable for applications where the spoken words of the user have to be identified by the computer. Such applications require machine learning techniques.

Machine learning techniques include the genetic algorithms and model-based methods. Some of the commonly used ones are neural networks, support vector machines (SVMs), and the hidden Markov model (HMM). Although earlier implementation was highly dependent on the speed of speech, more recent developments have overcome such shortcomings with the use of time warping techniques. However, the common implementation of these requires the assumption that all the relevant features of speech are input at one time to the system. Such assumptions may be suitable if the user is speaking individual characters. These also have applications in biometrics, where the identity of the speaker is being determined, or for emotive applications, where the emotion has to be identified. The HMM follows the flow of the features and the relationship of features as they progress over time, and is now routinely used for speech recognition applications.

9.11 Artificial neural networks

The classification of stationary speech features can be achieved by supervised learning techniques. This can be achieved using statistics as well as neural networks. Among the statistical techniques, the regression method and the Euclidian distances are the most popular methods for finding relationships between variables. There has been a lot of work done by various researchers in the use of artificial neural networks (ANNs) in the field of speech classification.

Neural networks have the capability to recognize, classify, convert, and learn patterns using examples of the data. Pattern recognition refers to the categorization of input data into identifiable classes by recognizing significant features or attributes of the data. The main advantage of choosing the neural networks for classification of surface electromyography (SEMG) data is that they can be used to solve difficult problems where the description of data is not computable. The major strength of ANNs is the fact that there is no need for any particular assumption of any statistical distributions and independence of input features. In addition, ANNs can be trained in such a way that a network exhibits discriminate properties. Unlike discriminate analysis in statistics, ANN does not require the linearity assumption and can be applied to nonlinearly separable classes.

The advantage of the use of neural networks is the ability of the network to determine the input–output relationship even when the relationship is not expressible by deterministic or statistical means. An advantage of the back propagation network is that, with the appropriate choice of momentum and training parameters, it avoids the local minimum and searches for an error surface along the gradient in order to minimize the error criteria. ANN can be trained for near real-time classification of speech and provide the user with necessary feedback to make required corrections.

Appropriate use of neural networks requires the normalization of the input features and the selection of its parameters. The size of the input to the ANN is dependent on the length of the feature vector, and the output is based on the number of outputs the ANN is trained to identify. There is no definite technique to select the size of hidden layers and number of hidden layers, but it is generally accepted that the number of neurons in the hidden layer are proportional to the complexity of the data set. The other important property of the ANN that has to be selected for the application includes the choice of training algorithm. There are also a number of parameters that require user selection (such as the acceptable error during training, maximum number of epochs during training, the threshold function for the output) and factors such as learning rate and momentum that determine the size of the steps and the likelihood of the network getting trained to a local rather than a global minima point.

9.11.1 Support vector machine

SVMs are a set of related supervised learning methods used for classification and regression. SVMs are used in a variety of fields like text classification, bioinformatics, handwriting recognition, and image analysis. SVMs are nonlinear machine learning algorithms, and have been used extensively for various audio, visual, clinical, and other applications. SVMs are suitable for regression and prediction and they require to be trained based on examples without requiring the user to define the relationship between the various factors. It is suitable for situations where examples of the different categories are available. During the training phase, the system identifies suitable weights that describe the complex relationship of the multiple factors and the categories, such as disease and case.

9.11.2 Hidden Markov model

A model that describes the possible sequence of events in context of the current condition is referred to as the Markov model. It provides the contextual information of the current sequence based on the previous sequence. HMM is a statistical Markov model with unobserved or hidden states and in the simplest form, considered to be a dynamic Bayesian network. HMM is considered in the family of nonlinear filtering and was developed by Baum et al. [4].

When all the states are known, the Markov models are modeled by state transition probabilities. In HMM, the state is not directly visible, but the output that is dependent on the state is visible. Each state has a probability distribution over the possible output tokens. Therefore, the sequence of these tokens generated by an HMM is based on the sequence of these states. Thus, the state sequence through which the model passes is hidden but not to the parameters of the model. HMM is especially known for its application in temporal pattern recognition where the properties are nonstationary, and some of those applications are speech, handwriting, gesture recognition, part-of-speech tagging, musical score following, partial discharges, and bioinformatics.

9.11.2.1 User benefits
Automatic speech and speaker recognition have been benefiting users from all walks of life, and have provided significant enhancement to the capabilities of people who lack the ability to use their hands. The technology has been extensively applied for a range of applications for able-bodied people and people with disabilities.

Automatic speaker recognition is widely used in the banking sector and organizations such as law-enforcement police force and social security that need to identify the speaker or confirm the identity of an individual. With the growth in telephone banking and use of telephone-based access for a range of services, machine-based identification of the speaker is extremely important, both for the speaker and for the organization.

Converting speech to commands is now routinely occurring. Although speech-based typing has been in many commercial applications and software, it is the need for hands-free telephone and GPS control in the car due to the safety concerns that necessitated the biggest single use of ASR algorithms. While the systems are still being improved to overcome shortcomings such as background noise, the advantage of automobile-based speech recognition is that modern cars are relatively low noise and often have only a single speaker, with stable acoustics between the driver and the microphone. This, along with the development of smarter and faster mobile phones, has made automobile-based speech recognition the most successful application.

Automatic speech analysis techniques are also employed for a range of other applications including converting speech to text. Such systems are now routinely being used by doctors to transcribe their patient interviews in order to generate the records. The technology is also regularly used by people who perform data-entry, a task that otherwise becomes very monotonous and can lead to errors during typing.

People who have suffered spinal cord injury and others who are unable to use their hands to type can use their speech instead. In the age of the Internet, this is very useful, as it provides them the ability to control their computer for performing Web browsing. Other applications are the use of speech to control devices such as wheelchairs, lighting, or curtains. Thus, someone who is unable to walk or use their hands is able to give verbal commands to manage their room facilities, or to command their mobility devices.

One of the more recent applications is the machine-based application identifying the emotions of the speaker. This can be used in computer games, interaction with robotic toys, and to identify psychological distress of a speaker to a helpline. Machine-based emotions identification of the speaker is helpful in determining the complexity of a computer game to make the games more interactive and for maintaining the appropriate level of challenge for the user. The developments of robotic toys that identify the emotions of the user are now routinely used for children and the elderly, with Japan leading the research. Identifying people who are distressed is becoming very important, especially with large number of services being telephone-based and having machine-based answering facilities.

9.12 Limitations in current systems

Humans are able to understand speech in complex environments even when there is high level of background noise or music or there are multiple speakers. Audio-based speech recognition is important but is not the only aspect of speech that we use to recognize speech, the speaker, or the emotions of the speaker. We have two ears, which are referred to as our binaural capabilities, and this gives us the ability to identify the spatial location of the source. We also use visual data, and numerous studies have shown that visualization of the speaker's mouth is an important aspect of our ability to understand speech in very noisy environments, such as music venues.

Over the past 20 years, with improved computational power and significant development in signal processing and classification techniques, speech-based systems are now robust and reliable. Speech-based systems are now routinely used for data entry, computer dictation, interacting with robotic devices, dialing telephone numbers, commanding devices inside a house, for speaker identification over the telephone, controlling vehicles, and for recognizing emotionally distressed people over the phone. These systems are now reasonably robust and are not very sensitive to background noise and differences between different microphones. However, they are sensitive to the presence of other people who are speaking in the background. Current systems require that the speaker be the only person speaking. This can be highly limiting and there is a need for the system to separate the audio of different speakers.

Recent developments have made the ASR robust and reliable; there are also many shortcomings in the current systems and that is why there is need for significant improvements. Some of the shortcomings are spatial localization of the speaker, background noise reduction, and separation of sounds from different sources. There is also the need for obtaining the context of the speech and integration of audio-based speech recognition with visual speech systems.

9.12.1 Recent developments

Improving ASR is being investigated by research teams around the world. Although some of this research is specific to a language or region, there are a number of generic topics that are being explored such as source separation, speaker localization, and audio–visual fusion. These are explained in the next sections.

9.12.1.1 Speaker source separation

In most real applications, the sources with temporal overlap, spectral or temporal filtering are not suitable. Consider a cocktail party, where there are number of speakers, and while the listeners who are embedded in the party are able to understand what is being spoken, an outsider to the party who is listening to the party using a microphone is unable to understand what is being spoken. This problem is often referred to as the blind source problem.

Blind source separation techniques have been developed since around 1995 [5,6]. One powerful blind source separation technique is an independent component analysis (ICA) [7,8]. It is based on the use of multiple recordings, where the number of sources is the same as the number of microphones. The separation of the different speakers does not require the speakers to have dissimilar features. The system assumes that the sources are independent of each other, and signals from different sources often get mixed during recording. Often it is required to separate the original signals, and there is little information available about the original signals.

An example is the cocktail party problem. Even if there is no (limited) information available about the original signals or the mixing matrix, it is possible to separate the original signals using ICA under certain conditions. ICA is an iterative technique that estimates the statistically independent source signals from a given set of their linear combinations. The process involves determining the mixing matrix. The independent sources could be audio signals (such as speech, voice, and music) or bioelectric signals.

If the mixing process is assumed to be linear, it can be expressed as

$$x = As$$

where $x = x_1(t), ..., x_n(t)$ is the recordings; $s = s_1(t), ..., s_n(t)$ is the original signals; and A is the $n \times n$ mixing matrix of real numbers.

This mixing matrix and each of the original signals are unknown. To separate the recordings to the original signals, the task is to estimate an unmixing matrix W so that $s = Wx$. For this purpose, ICA relies strongly on the statistical independence of the sources. This technique iteratively estimates the unmixing matrix using the maximization of independence of the sources as the cost function.

Signals $s = s_1(t), ..., s_n(t)$ are statistically independent if the joint probability density of those components can be expressed as a multiplication of their marginal probability density. It is important to observe the distinction between independence and uncorrelatedness, since decorrelation can always be performed by transforming the signals with a whitening matrix V to get the identity covariance matrix I. Independent signals are always uncorrelated but uncorrelated signals are not always independent. But in the case of Gaussian signals, uncorrelatedness implies independence. Transforming of a Gaussian signal with any orthogonal unmixing matrix or transform results in another Gaussian signal, and thus the original signals cannot be separated. Hence, Gaussian signals are forbidden for ICA. Thus, the key of independent component estimation is measuring the non-Gaussianity of the signals.

There are several measures of non-Gaussianity that can be used. The classical one is Kurtosis value or fourth-order cumulant. This value is zero, negative, and positive for Gaussian, sub-Gaussian, and super-Gaussian data, respectively. The absolute value of Kurtosis is frequently used since it will be either zero or positive, and will reach its maximum value when the signal is independent. Furthermore, Gaussianity also implies the degree of randomness of a signal and is related to the information content of a signal. The less random signal (more structured signal) carries less information than the random one and vice versa. The Gaussian signal is the most random signal among other signals and therefore it has the potential for the largest possible information content.

Due to the central limit theorem, information content and mutual information of $x = x_1(t), \ldots, x_n(t)$ must be higher than that of $s = s_1(t), \ldots, s_n(t)$. Therefore, entropy (a measure of information content of a signal) can also be used as another measure of non-Gaussianity of a signal. Examples of ICA algorithms based on non-Gaussianity maximization are the Infomax algorithm by Bell and Sejnowski [7,8] and fast ICA algorithm by Hyvarinen [6]. The detailed derivations of the corresponding learning rules of those algorithms are available in these papers. These rules or conditions are listed next. The successful separation of the original signals is dependent on the fulfillment of these conditions [7].

- The sources must be statistically independent.
- The sources must have non-Gaussian distributions. However, the work by McKeown [9] has demonstrated that ICA will still work properly if not more than one of the independent sources is Gaussian.
- The number of available recordings must be at least the same as the number of the independent sources.
- The recorded signals must be a (approximately) linear combination of the independent sources.
- There should be no (little) noise common to the sources and there should be no (minimal) delay between the signals of the different sources in the recordings.

Although ICA has demonstrated success in the ability to separate signals, the output of ICA suffers from numerous ambiguities. Review of the publications that report the use of ICA for SEMG filtering and separation reveals only one research article [10] that has acknowledged these shortcomings. The shortcomings are

- The order of the independent components cannot be fixed and this may change for each estimate.
- The amplitude and sign of the independent components cannot be determined. Although the relative amplitude within each signal is correctly estimated, relative amplitude between different signals cannot be estimated using ICA.

In most applications such as the cocktail party problem, these are not serious problems. The supervisor is able to identify the different sources and determine the quality of the separation by listening to the sounds. When dealing with signals such as bio-electric signals, the order of signals may be important as would be the absolute value of the signal magnitude, and the supervisor may not be able to identify the order in any other way. Further, it is also important to have an objective measure of the quality of the separation as the technique used for sound is no longer valid. This is often difficult as the signals are obviously unknown and the purpose of the study would be to identify the possible physiological abnormalities based on the signals. Thus, it is important to determine the quality of separation ahead of the experiments. As this is also difficult when using real signals, one easier alternative is to determine how well the signals match with the necessary conditions for ICA and to test the separation using synthetic signals to determine the efficacy of the separation. Successful separation could then be extrapolated to the real signals.

As noted earlier, the signals that can be separated need to be non-Gaussian and independent. For the purpose of applying ICA to bioelectric recordings, there is a need to determine the conditions under which the bioelectric signals can be considered as independent and non-Gaussian, and the mixing matrix can be considered to be stationary and linear. This chapter analyzes the conditions under which the bioelectric signals can be considered independent with a linear and stationary mixing matrix.

Although standard ICA requires that the number of signals be less than or equal to the number of recordings, some researchers have attempted to overcome this limitation by developing techniques to separate overcomplete (sources are more than recordings) recordings [11–13]. In some of these papers, the quality of separation has not been objectively measured. The concern with the technique proposed by Zibulevsky is that it is based on the assumption that the signals are sparse. This is not always possible, and in some cases this may require preprocessing of the data.

The authors have not been able to identify published research where a suitable measure of quality of separation has been reported. This chapter has proposed a measure for the quality of separation. The measure requires determining the closeness of the mixing and the unmixing matrices using synthetic signals prior to the use of ICA for bioelectric signals can be established.

9.12.1.2 Audio and visual fusion

In this chapter, visual-based speech recognition techniques have been described. Such systems are suitable for a small range of speech commands. However, fusing the visual with the audio has been shown to make speech recognition more robust and reliable. Research teams [14,15] are attempting to develop speech recognition systems that take the advantage of the presence of a camera and microphone on many consumer devices such as mobile phones.

References

1. KALMAN RE. A new approach to linear filtering and prediction problems. Transactions of the ASME. *Journal of Basic Engineering.* 1960: 35–45.

2. LAURITZEN S. Time series analysis in 1880: A discussion of contributions made by T. N. Thiele. *International Statistics Review.* 1981:49, 319–331.

3. SWERLING P. Modern state estimation methods from the viewpoint of the method of least squares. *IEEE Transactions on Automatic Control.* 1971:AC-16, 707–719.

4. BAUM LE, PETRIE T, GEORGE S, NORMAN W. A maximization technique occurring in the statistical analysis of probabilistic functions of Markov chains. *Annals of Mathematical Statistics* 1970:41(1), 164–171.

5. COMON P. Independent component analysis, a new concept? *Signal Processing* 1994:36(3), 287–314.

6. HYVARINEN A. Fast and robust fixed-point algorithms for independent component analysis. *IEEE Transactions on Neural Networks* 1999:10(3), 626–634.

7. BELL AJ, SEJNOWSKI TJ. An information-maximization approach to blind separation and blind deconvolution. *Neural Computation.* 1995:7(6), 1129–1159.

8. BELL AJ, SEJNOWSKI TJ. The "independent components" of natural scenes are edge filters. *Vision Research* 1997:37(23), 3327–3338.

9. McKEOWN MJ, JUNG TP, MAKEIG S, BROWN G, KINDERMANN SS, LEE TW, SEJNOWSKI TJ. Spatially independent activity patterns in functional MRI data during the Stroop color-naming task. *Proceedings of the National Academy of Sciences, USA* 1998:95(3), 803–810. 104

10. GRECO A, COSTANTINO D, MORABITO FC, VERSACI M. A Morlet wavelet classification technique for ICA filtered sEMG experimental data. In *Proceedings of the International Joint Conference on Neural Networks, 2003* 2003:1, 166–171.

11. BOFILL P, ZIBULEVSKY M. Blind separation of more sources than mixtures using sparsity of their short-time Fourier transform. In *Proceedings of the ICA 2000* 2000: 87–92.

12. LEE TW, BELL AJ, LAMBERT RH. Blind separation of delayed and convolved sources. *Advances in Neural Information Processing Systems* 1997:9, 758–764.

13. ZIBULEVSKY M, PEARLMUTTER BA. Blind source separation by sparse decomposition in a signal dictionary. *Neural Computation* 2001:13(4), 863–882.

14. LU H, BRUSH AJB, PRIYANTHA B, KARLSON AK, LIU J. Speaker sense: Energy efficient unobtrusive speaker identification on mobile phones. *Pervasive Computing, Lecture Notes in Computer Science* 2011:6696, 188–205.

15. ZHANG Z, HERSHEY J. Fusing array microphone and stereo vision for improved computer interfaces (Microsoft Research Technical Report MSR-TR-2005–174). Microsoft Corporation, Redmond, WA. Smart Technologies, Incorporated 2005.

CHAPTER TEN

Lip movement for human–computer interface

Abstract

Speech-based computer control has found a large number of applications and users employing their natural speech communication and manipulation skills. However, speech-impaired people and people in very noisy environments are unable to avail of this technology. Silent speech-based technologies have been developed to overcome this shortcoming. Silent speech-based assistive technologies are important for users with difficulty to vocalize and provide the ability for such users to give commands and control computers without making a sound. These technologies are generally based on analyzing the movement of the mouth, or the throat, or guttural airflow analysis. This chapter describes the technologies and evaluates two technologies that have been developed for recognizing facial movements: facial muscle activity and video of the mouth. It investigates the classification power of mouth videos in identifying English vowels and consonants, and the impact of language on the outcome, by comparing the difference between native and foreign languages. The effect of feedback to the user who uses such a system is also discussed.

10.1 Introduction: History and applications

Facial expressions and movements of the lips are generally encoded in speech, offer rich information, and are suitable for complex commands to a computer [1]. Speech-based human–computer interface (HCI) utilizes a natural ability of the human user and has the potential for computer control to be rich, natural, and effortless. Such systems have the potential to assist people who are unable to use their hands due to disease or special circumstances [2]. Over the past two decades, these systems have become relatively commonplace and offer reliable options for the users to substitute for a keyboard and perform tasks, such as typing or controlling machines. Speech recognition systems can be deployed in applications such as vehicle control systems [3], assistive technology (AT), security and surveillance systems, and telephony [4].

Speech-based systems have grown into a fully independent industry, with applications such as hands-free control of devices in a car, computer games, assistive technologies, and emotional interaction with robotic devices. Users of all ages benefit from automatic speech recognition technologies. However, these technologies have significant shortcomings and require a user to speak clearly and audibly, require the background noise to be significantly lower than the speech command, and require the acoustics to be remain unchanged. However, there are a number of situations where these conditions are not possible, such as:

- The person suffers from voice disorders that may be due to the air passage from the lungs. This may be a result of muscle weakness or dysarthria resulting in lack of speech and suitable airflow from the lungs.
- Noise from the background, such as traffic noise.
- The need to speak softly in open offices.
- Special situations such as during defense situations.

Advantages of a voiceless speech-based system are (1) recognition is not affected by background noise, or changes in acoustic conditions, and (2) it does not require the user to verbalize the speech and make a sound. Our ability to speak utilizes a number of complex movements such as movement of the palate, throat, and lips; control of the rate of airflow; and use of our nostrils. Recognizing voiceless speech can be done using nonacoustic modalities, such as visual [5], recording of vocal cords movements [6], mechanical sensing of facial movement and movement of palate, recording of facial muscle activity [7], facial plethysmogram, and measuring the intraoral pressure. When we use a single modality to recognize speech or oral commands, there is an inherent loss of information and the available vocabulary has to be significantly reduced.

Each of the voiceless speech recognition techniques has inherent limitations, such as the need for placing sensors inside the mouth or on the skin. The limitations are also associated with reduced and limited vocabulary, and the need for significant training of the user. From the literature, the most effective methods that have significant vocabulary and provide reliability without being invasive are (1) visual recognition of the movement of the lips using the video of the mouth and (2) recognition of the lip and mouth movement by recording the facial muscle activity (surface electromyography, SEMG).

The visual recognition is effective because it does not require the user to have any sensor placed on the face, and the video camera may be placed in a convenient location. However, it suffers from the disadvantage of being usable only in the presence of suitable lighting conditions, and unsuitable for being used in dark. An SEMG-based system has the advantage of being usable without requiring light, but suffers from the need to have metal electrodes in contact with the face of the user and is susceptible to the factors such as sweat on the skin. One common difficulty in the use of these technologies is the dependence on factors such as culture and language and differences between individuals.

This chapter discusses these two modalities based on video and SEMG signal in detail. It describes the technical details of these modalities and discusses some of the challenges and shortcomings, such as the native language and future directions based on the current research. It focuses on the identification of phonemes, because a phoneme-based system can be extended for word recognition by concatenating the phonemes to form words.

10.2 Current technologies

10.2.1 Video-based speech analyzer

A vision-based technique to recognize speech requires a combination of hardware that will record the movement of the lips and software that will identify the phoneme. A microphone may also be required to train the system and link the video of the mouth with the audio. In this section, visual speech recognition (VSR) developed to recognize English vowels and consonants based on the visible facial movement has been described.

The video recording is a relatively straightforward task, and most low-resolution cameras are suitable for this task. The movement of the mouth does not require high spatial or temporal resolution, and a portable, inexpensive commercially available camera is sufficient. The next stage of a typical VSR

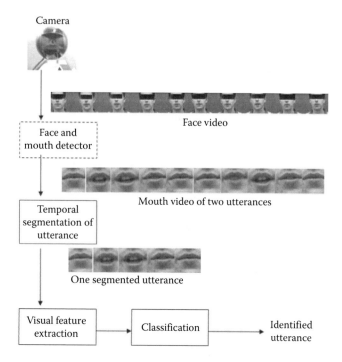

FIGURE 10.1 Block diagram of the visual speech recognition technique reported in the literature.

technique requires the analysis of the video to identify the unvoiced speech, and this consists of three stages: (1) video processing for facial motion segmentation, (2) visual feature extraction, and (3) classification. There are numerous visual speech features that may be extracted from the videos [10–12] and they can be broadly categorized into shape-based, pixel-based, and motion-based features. A block diagram of a VSR system is shown in Figure 10.1.

This section investigates the viability of a VSR technique based on motion features extracted using spatial-temporal templates (STTs) in English phoneme recognition. A visual speech model based on the Moving Picture Experts Group 4 (MPEG-4) standard has been used to map the consonants to different facial movements.

10.2.1.1 Video processing to segment facial movement The first step in VSR is to determine when the user wants to speak. For this purpose, the system needs to undertake temporal segmentation and identify when the speaker begins to actively open the mouth, which is the cue to start to speak.

A motion-identification-based segmentation technique is required to identify the start and completion of movement. One method that has been proposed is to represent the movement using a 2D grayscale image (STTs) [5]. An STT shows where and when facial movements occur in the image sequence [13].

One technique to generate STTs is by using the accumulative image difference approach. Difference of frames (DOFs) is obtained. The zero intensity DOF indicates that there is no movement during that period. DOFs are obtained by performing the image subtraction of successive frames on the video of the speaker. These DOFs are binarized using an optimum threshold value, which may be determined by the supervisor or by statistical analysis and identifying the knee point of the images. Similarly, the delimiters for identifying the start and stop of the conversation may be inserted by the supervisor based on statistical analysis.

The temporal location of the DOF is inserted in the STT by multiplying the intensity of the DOF with a ramp function of time. The intensity of the STT at the start of the motion of the identified segment becomes less, while those STTs near the end of the segment become high. The intensity value of the STT at pixel location (x, y) of the tth frame is defined by

$$STT_t(x,y) = \max \bigcup_{t=1}^{N-1} B_t(x,y) \times t \qquad (10.1)$$

where N is the total number of frames of the video and $B_t(x,y)$ represents the binarized version of the DOF of frame t. In Equation 10.1, $B_t(x, y)$ is multiplied with a linear ramp of time to implicitly encode the temporal information of the facial motions into the STT. By computing the STT values for all the pixels, the coordinates (x, y) of the image sequence using Equation 10.1 will produce a grayscale image (STT) where the brightness of the pixels indicates the recency of motion in the image sequence.

10.2.1.2 Issues related to the facial movement segmentation

An STT is a view-sensitive motion representation technique. Therefore, the STT generated from the sequence of images is dependent on factors:

- *The angle*—The system works best when the position of the speaker's mouth and face is normal to the camera's optical axis.

- *Scale or distance*—The distance of the speaker's mouth from the camera; this needs to be fixed, and a change in the distance changes the scale/size of the mouth in the frame.

- *Translation*—The camera is fixed with respect to the mouth, and small movement of the head of the speaker can lead to an error.

The STT's representative features need to be rotation, translation, and scale invariant so that the system is robust and reliable. Wavelet transform is a useful technique to represent an image. However, the discrete wavelet transform (DWT) is translation variant [14] where a small shift of the image in the space domain will yield very different wavelet coefficients. The translation sensitivity of DWT is caused by the aliasing effect that occurs due to the downsampling of the image along the rows and columns [15]. One such method is the use of discrete stationary wavelet transform (SWT). The SWT representation of the STT is insensitive to small variations of the mouth and lip movement. SWT restores the translation invariance of the signal by omitting the downsampling process of DWT and results in redundancies.

Two-dimensional SWT at level 1 when applied on the STT produces a spatial-frequency representation of the STT. The 2D SWT is implemented by applying 1D SWT along the rows of the image followed by 1D SWT along the columns of the image. SWT decomposition of the MHI generates four images: approximation (LL), horizontal detail coefficients (LH), vertical detail coefficients (HL), and diagonal detail coefficients (HH) through iterative filtering using low- and high-pass filters. The approximate image is the smoothed version of the STT, contains the trend information, and has the highest energy content; while LH, HL, and HH contain the detail and represent the fluctuations of the pixel intensity in the horizontal, vertical, and diagonal directions. The detailed coefficients carry the noise and generally correspond to isolated changes, and the trend corresponds to the movement of a complete object that has a connected contour. Thus, for this work, the approximate coefficient images are required and used for further analysis.

Zernike moments represent the image into region-based features and these are rotation, translation, and scale invariant/insensitive. These are rich in information, and yet compact and thus suitable for representing the STT.

10.2.1.3 Extraction of visual speech features

Zernike moments are image feature descriptors that are commonly used for representing images [16,17]. These have been demonstrated to outperform other image moments, such as geometric moments, Legendre moments, and complex moments in terms of robustness to image noise, and are suitable for reducing information redundancy and provide sufficient information for image representation [18]. The proposed technique uses Zernike moments as visual speech features to represent the SWT approximate image of the STT.

Zernike moments are computed by projecting the image function $f(x, y)$ onto the orthogonal Zernike polynomial V_{nl} of order n with repetition l is defined within a unit circle (i.e., $x^2 + y^2 \leq 1$) as follows:

$$V_{nl}(\rho,\theta) = R_{nl}(\rho)e^{-jl\theta}; \quad \hat{J} = \sqrt{-1} \tag{10.2}$$

where R_{nl} is the real-valued radial polynomial.

Zernike moments provide rotational invariant features [16] and are computationally inexpensive, making these suitable for real-time operations. The absolute value of Zernike moments is invariant to the rotational changes of mouth in the videos [5]. These moments are orthogonal V_{nl} [18]. $|l| \leq n$ and $(n - |l|)$ is even, and thus provide a set of independent features, making these suitable for classification.

Based on the aforementioned properties of Zernike moments, the image needs to be within a unit circle that is centered at the origin. Thus, the wavelet-transformed approximate 1 images of STT need to be scaled such that it is within a unit circle centered at the origin such that the unit circle is bounded by the square of the scaled version of the image. The center of the image is considered as the origin of the axis, and the pixel coordinates are then mapped to the range of the unit circle, that is, $x^2 + y^2 \leq 1$, and this is shown in Figure 10.2. Zernike moments transform the square image function $(f(x, y))$ which is in terms of the x–y axes to a circular image function $(f(\rho,\theta))$ which is in terms of the i–j axes.

The accuracy of identifying a specific movement of the mouth requires a higher number of independent features that will be representing the STT. For this purpose, higher-order Zernike moments are required. However, this inherently increases the size of the features, makes it sensitive to noise, and increases the computational complexity. There is a need to identify the most suitable number of Zernike moments to be selected. Experiments have revealed that 49 Zernike moments that comprise of zeroth-order moments up to 12th-order moments are suitable, and provide sufficient sensitivity and specificity to identify the consonant [19].

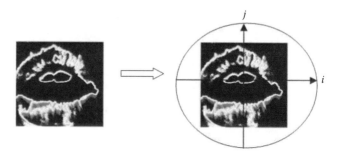

FIGURE 10.2   The square-to-circular transformation of the SWT approximation of STT.

10.2.2 Speech recognition based on facial muscle activity

Speech can be parameterized in terms of phonemes, the combination of which forms the spoken characters and words. The required shape of the mouth and lips for the utterance of the phonemes is achieved by the movement and maintained shape of the mouth, and this is achieved by facial muscles [20,21]. The electrical activity of the muscles can be recorded from the surface and used to identify the shape and movement of the mouth.

The recording of the electrical activity of the muscles is referred to as the electromyogram or EMG. The EMG corresponding to the facial muscles has the information associated with the muscle contraction shape and movement of the face, and has been found to be suitable for identifying the unvoiced phonemes. Unlike a video-based system, which is suitable for consonants, this is more suitable for identifying the maintained shape of the mouth, and, thus, suitable for vowels. This may also be suitable for identifying commands to the machine or the computer. The system has the advantage that it does not require light and is insensitive to the lighting conditions. However, it requires an electrical contact between the facial skin and the recording device.

To understand the functioning of this method, the production of speech and the muscles that produce speech will be discussed in the following sections.

10.2.2.1 Face movement related to speech   The face can communicate a variety of information, including subjective emotion, communicative intent, and cognitive appraisal. Effective speech and emotional display require specific movement of the mouth and precise muscle control. One difficulty with speech identification using facial movement and shape is the temporal variation when the user is uttering sounds that have complex time and spectral envelopes. With the intra- and intersubject variation in the speed of speaking and the length of each sound, it is difficult to determine a suitable window length and to identify suitable signal features that are robust.

Other difficulties arise from the need for segmentation and the identification of the start and end of movement. Root mean square (RMS) is an effective technique to identify the envelope of the signal, and conducting the statistical analysis of this provides the suitable threshold for identifying the temporal location of each activity.

10.2.2.2 Features of SEMG An SEMG is the noninvasive recording of the muscle activity. It can be recorded from the surface using electrodes that are in contact with the skin and located close to the muscle to be studied. The SEMG is a gross indicator of the muscle activity and is used to identify the force of muscle contraction, associated movement, and posture [22]. Using an SEMG-based system, Chan et al. [23] demonstrated the presence of speech information in facial myoelectric signals. Kumar et al. [24] demonstrated the use of an SEMG to identify unspoken sounds under controlled conditions.

It is relatively simple to identify the start and the end of the muscle activity related to the vowel, because the muscle activity at the start and the end is much greater than the activity in the middle. During the phase when the mouth cavity shape is maintained static, such as corresponding to the formation of the vowel, the muscle activity is small, and this leads to difficulties such as a poor signal-to-noise ratio.

While developing a system to recognize voiceless speech, the variation in the intersubject leads to the need for customization of the system to each user. Variations, such as in the speed and style of utterance of the vowel, can lead to very significant variations in the STT. To overcome this, the recordings can be normalized and the recommended normalization factor can be the integration of the RMS of the SEMG from the start till the end of the utterance of the vowel.

10.3 User requirements

10.3.1 Video-based voiceless speech recognition

A video-based voiceless speech recognition system is suitable for people who produce suitable and repeatable facial and mouth movement corresponding to specific speech, but are unable to produce sufficient sound intensity. The implementation of such a system will require sufficient background lighting as well as the ability of the user to have a headphone-mounted camera to record the video of the lips. Experiments to test such a system are described in Section 10.4.1.

10.3.2 EMG-based voiceless speech recognition

An EMG-based voiceless speech recognition system is suitable for the people who have healthy control on their facial muscles. The people who would benefit from such a system would be able to perform the movement of the mouth but unable to produce quality sound. This may be due to conditions, such as lack of control of their larynx, poor airflow pressure, or the inability to produce sound because they are in an open office or in special situations.

The system requires the recording of the SEMG from the facial muscles, and this necessitates the use of surface-mounted electrodes on the face. Thus, it is necessary that the user is comfortable with the presence of such electrodes on the face for this technology. Experiments to test such a system are described in Section 10.4.2.

10.4 Example of voiceless speech recognition systems

This chapter gives examples of two voiceless speech recognition techniques. The first is video-based and the second is EMG-based. Both of these have their strengths and shortcomings, and the choice would be based on the application. In the following sections, the implementation of the technology, the experiments conducted to test it, and the results are provided.

10.4.1 Video data acquisition and processing

Video data was recorded using an inexpensive, low-resolution Web camera in a typical office setting. This was done to test the practicality of such a system for voiceless communication. The ambient lighting conditions and complex and varying background tests the robustness of the visual voiceless system. The audio noise helps put the application in perspective for the user.

The camera was fixed to a mouthpiece that was worn by the user (Figure 10.3), and was focused on the mouth region of the speaker. Although such a system did not stop small movements, the translation, rotation, and scale changes were only small. The following were the factors that were considered during the recordings:

- Camera resolution and frame rate
- Window size of the camera

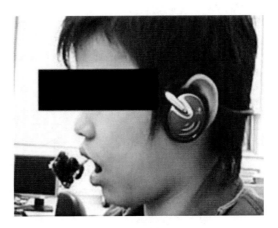

FIGURE 10.3 A visual voiceless speech recognition system. (From Yau WC, Video analysis of mouth movement using motion templates for computer-based lip-reading, Doctoral dissertation, RMIT University, Melbourne, Australia, 2008. Available at: https://researchbank.rmit.edu.au/view/rmit:6864/Yau.pdf. With permission.)

- View angle of the camera
- Background
- Ambient lighting

The technology was tested by conducting experiments with volunteer subjects in accordance with the human ethics approval that was obtained prior to the experiments. The experiments were to test the visual speech recognition technique. Consonants that form the viseme model of English consonants according to the MPEG-4 standard were used in the experiment: m, v, T, t, g, tS, s, n, r, A, e, I, Q, U.

One hundred eighty video files with the resolution of 240×240 pixels were recorded and stored as true color (.AVI) files. The frame rate of the AVI files was 30 frames per second. One STT was generated from each AVI file. SWT at level 1 using the Haar wavelet was applied on the STTs and the approximate image (LL) was used for analysis. Forty-nine Zernike moments have been used as features.

10.4.2 Visual speech recognizer The classification accuracies of the HMM trained using visual features are tabulated in Table 10.1. The average recognition rate of the proposed vision-based system is 88.2%. The results indicate that the proposed technique based on motion features is suitable for the recognition of English phonemes.

Table 10.1 Mean recognition rates of the visual speech recognizer based on viseme model of MPEG-4 standard

Viseme	Recognition rate (%)
m	95
v	90
T	70
t	80
g	85
tS	95
s	95
n	40
r	100
A:	100
e	100
I	95
Q	95
U	95

Based on the results, it can be said that the proposed technique is highly accurate for vowels' classification using the motion features. An average success rate of 97% is achieved in recognizing vowels. The classification accuracies of consonants are slightly lower. Table 10.2 shows the differences in error rates for vowels and consonants. The results indicate that the consonants are less distinguishable than vowels using visual speech features.

The classification errors can be attributed to the inability of vision-based techniques to capture the occluded movements of speech articulators, such as the glottis, velum, and tongue. For example, the tongue movement in the mouth cavity is either partially or completely not visible (occluded by the teeth) in the video data during the pronunciation of alveolar and dental sounds such as /t/, /T/, and /n/.

Table 10.2 Mean recognition rates for English vowels and consonants

Vowels/consonants	Recognition rate
Vowels	97
Consonants	83.33

The STTs of /t/, /T/, and /n/ do not contain the information of the occluded tongue movements. This is a possible reason for the higher error rates of 20%, 30%, and 60% for these three consonants as compared to the average error rate of 12% for all visemes. Consonantal sounds with similar facial movements may cause ambiguities that affect the performance of a visual speech recognizer.

To compare the results of the proposed approach with other related work is inappropriate due to the different video corpus and recognition tasks used. In a similar visual-only speech recognition task (based on the 14 visemes of MPEG-4 standard) reported by Arjunan et al. [25], a similar error rate was obtained using shape-based features (geometric measures of the lip) extracted from static images. Nevertheless, the errors made in our proposed visual system using motion features are different as compared to the errors reported by Foo and Dong [26]. This indicates that complementary information exists in the static and dynamic features of visual speech.

For example, our proposed system has a much lower error rate in identifying visemes /m/, /t/, and /r/ by using the facial movement features as compared to the results of Arjunan et al. [25]. This shows that motion features are better in representing phones, which involve distinct facial movements (such as the bilabial movements of /m/). The static features of Arjunan et al. [25] yield better results in classifying visemes with ambiguous or occluded motion of the speech articulators such as /n/. The results demonstrate that a computationally inexpensive system can easily be developed on a digital signal processor chip for silent speech-based AT.

10.4.3 Experiments using facial muscle activity signals

Experiments were conducted to test the performance of the proposed speech recognition from facial SEMG for two different languages, German and English. The experiments were approved by the Human Experiments Ethics Committee of the university. In controlled experiments, participants were asked to speak while their SEMG were recorded. The SEMG recordings were visually observed, and all recordings with any artifact—typically due to loose electrodes or movement—were discarded.

During these recordings, the participants spoke three selected English vowels (/a/, /e/, /u/) and three selected German vowels (/a/, /i/, /u/). Each vowel was spoken separately such that there was a clear start and end of its utterance. The experiment was repeated 10 times for each language. A suitable resting time was given between each experiment. The participants were asked to vary their speaking speed and style to obtain a wide training set.

10.4.3.1 Facial EMG recording and preprocessing

The participants in the experiment were native speakers of German with English as their second language. Four-channel facial SEMG was recorded using the recommended recording guidelines [27]. A four-channel, portable, continuous recording MEGAWIN instrument (Mega Electronics, Finland) was used for this purpose. In this study, *four* facial muscles were selected: *zygomaticus major, depressor angulioris, masseter,* and *mentalis* [27]. The details of the experiment have been reported [19,25,28,29].

10.4.3.2 Data analysis

The first step in the analysis of the data was to identify the temporal location of the muscle activity. Moving RMS (MRMS) of the recorded signal with a threshold of 1 sigma of the signal was applied for windowing and identifying the start and the end of the active period [30]. A Window size of 20 samples corresponding to 10 ms has been shown to be suitable for computing the MRMS.

The next step was the integration of the MRMS of all the four channels and in the complete range of the speech, from the start until the end of the associated muscle activity. This provided a vector with four parameters, corresponding to the overall activity of the four channels for each vowel utterance. This data was normalized by computing a ratio of integrated MRMS of each channel with respect to channel 1. This ratio is indicative for the relative strength of contraction of the different muscles and reduces the impact of interexperimental variations.

10.4.3.3 Classification of visual and facial EMG features

For classification, the supervised neural network approach was used with the parameterized data, resulting in a vector for each utterance. The ANN consisted of two hidden layers with 20 nodes in both layers. Sigmoid function was used as the threshold decision. The ANN was trained with a gradient descent algorithm using a momentum with a learning rate of 0.05 to reduce the likelihood of local minima. Finally, the trained ANN was used to classify the test data. This entire process was repeated for each of the participants.

A random subsampling cross-validation method was used to determine the mean classification accuracy of the normalized features of the facial SEMG. The training and testing of different random subsamples using the ANN were repeated for different times. The final classification accuracy is the average of individual estimates.

10.5 Discussion: User benefits

Table 10.3 shows the ANN classification results on the test data using weight matrix generated during training for English vowels and for German vowels. These results indicate that the mean classification accuracy of the integral RMS values of the EMG signal yields a better recognition rate of vowels for three different participants, when the ANN classifier is trained individually. The results indicate that this technique can be used for the classification of vowels for the native and foreign language—in this case, English and German. This suggests that the system based on facial muscle activity is able to identify the differences between the styles of speaking of different people at different times for different languages.

The error rate in classification accuracy for a foreign language (English) is marginally higher compared with the native language (German). This is because the muscle pattern remains the same during the utterance of the native language and changes during the utterance of the foreign language. The variation is high for German vowels /a/, /i/ and English vowels /a/, /e/, and there is no variation for the vowel /u/ in both German and English language.

The results indicate that the proposed method using activities of facial muscles for identifying silently spoken vowels is technically feasible from the viewpoint of error in identification. The investigation reveals the suitability of the system for

Table 10.3 Mean classification errors for English and German vowels

| | Mean classification errors | | |
Vowel	Subject 1 (%)	Subject 2 (%)	Subject 3 (%)
English			
/a/	27	17	20
/e/	24	24	17
/u/	0	0	0
German			
/a/	14	17	17
/i/	4	20	24
/u/	0	0	0

English and German, and suggests that the system is feasible when used for people speaking their own native language as well as a foreign language.

The results also indicate that the system is not disturbed by the variation in the speed of utterance. The recognition accuracy is high when it is trained and tested for a dedicate user. Hence, such a system could be used by any individual user as a reliable HCI. This method has only been tested for limited vowels. The promising results obtained in the experiment indicate that facial muscle movement represents a suitable and reliable method for classifying vowels of single user without regard to speaking speed and style for different languages. It should be pointed out that the proposed technique based on facial muscle activity does not provide the flexibility of continuous speech, but for a limited dictionary of discrete phones, which is appropriate for simple voice-control-based AT systems. Furthermore, the results suggest that such a system is suitable and reliable for simple commands for HCI when it is trained for the user.

10.6 Summary

This chapter reported the feasibility of subauditory speech recognition approaches using two different modalities: (1) based on video data and (2) measurement of the facial muscle contraction using noninvasive SEMG [25,28]. The application of this includes the removal of any errors caused by the background acoustic noise or poor acoustics, and provides another option for human–computer-based assistive devices.

The SEMG system was tested for vowels in two languages and not consonants because vowels require stationary muscle contraction as compared to consonants making the automatic segmentation of the signal easier to implement. This highlights the limitations of the technology and suggests that for a complete system, there is the need for an alternate technique to identify the cues for segmenting the SEMG recordings.

The recognition accuracy for the SEMG-based system is high when it is trained and tested for a dedicated user in both German and English. This study also examines a vision-based technique to recognize English vowels and consonants. The experimental results of the visual approach demonstrate that the visual speech information can be used to reliably classify a set of English phonemes. One basic application for such a system is for a disabled user with speech impairment to give simple commands to a machine, which would be a helpful and typical application of AT.

The EMG-based investigation also compared the system based on the language the user was speaking in English and German. The results show that there was a significant difference in the recognition accuracy when the person spoke in their native language compared with the foreign tongue. This may be because people find it easier to repeat the same action they are very familiar with compared with the actions they have to train themselves with later.

The video-based system implementation shows that such a system is easy to implement using a camcorder fitted in place of the microphone of the headphones. The results demonstrate the strength of such a system, and with inexpensive and easy to obtain cameras, this has higher user acceptability. Such a system was also found suitable for a range of sounds including the consonants. The only shortcoming of such a system was the requirement of sufficient background lighting. With the availability of good quality cameras located on the smartphones and sufficient computing power, the implementation of such a system is achievable by simply having suitable software. However, to the knowledge of the authors, no such commercial system is available.

References

1. URSULA H, PIERRE P. Facial reactions to emotional facial expressions: Affect or cognition? *Cognition and Emotion* 1998:12(4), 509–531.
2. FENG J, SEARS A, KARAT C. A longitudinal evaluation of hands-free speech-based navigation during dictation. *International Journal of Human-Computer Studies* 2006:64, 553–569.
3. KUHN T, JAMEEL A, STUEMPFLE M, HADDADI A. Hybrid in-car speech recognition for mobile multimedia applications. In *IEEE Vehicular Technology Conference* 1999:3, 2009–2013.
4. STARKIE B. Programming spoken dialogs using grammatical inference. AI 2001: Advances in Artificial Intelligence: 14th International Joint Conference on Artificial Intelligence, Adelaide, Australia, 2001.
5. YAU WC, KUMAR DK, ARJUNAN SP. Visual speech recognition method using translation, scale and rotation invariant features. IEEE International Conference on Advanced Video and Signal based Surveillance, Sydney, Australia, 2006.
6. DIKSHIT PS, SCHUBERT RW. Electroglottograph as an additional source of information in isolated word recognition. In *Proceedings of the 14th Southern Biomedical Engineering Conference* 1995: 1–4.

7. ARJUNAN S, KUMAR DK, WEGHORN H, NAIK G. Facial muscle activity patterns for recognition of utterances in native and foreign language: Testing for its reliability and flexibility. In *Cross-Disciplinary Applications of Artificial Intelligence and Pattern Recognition: Advancing Technologies*, edited by V Mago, N Bhatia, 212–231. Information Science Reference, Hershey, PA, 2012.

8. POTAMIANOS G, NETI C, GRAVIER G, SENIOR AW. Recent advances in automatic recognition of audio-visual speech. In *Proceedings of the IEEE* 2003:91(9), 1306–1326.

9. HAZEN TJ. Visual model structures and synchrony constraints for audio-visual speech recognition. *IEEE Transactions on Audio, Speech, and Language Processing* 2006:14(3), 1082–1089.

10. PETAJAN ED. Automatic lip-reading to enhance speech recognition. In *IEEE Global Telecommunication Conference*, Atlanta, GA, pp. 265–272, 1984.

11. KAYNAK MN, QI Z, CHEOK AD, SENGUPTA K, CHUNG KC. Audio-visual modeling for bimodal speech recognition. In *IEEE Transactions on Systems, Man, and Cybernetics*, 2001:1, 181–186.

12. ADJOUDANI A, BENOIT C, LEVINE EP. On the integration of auditory and visual parameters in an HMM-based ASR. *Speechreading by Humans and Machines: Models, Systems, and Applications* 1996:150, 461–472.

13. BOBICK AF, DAVIS JW. The recognition of human movement using temporal templates. *IEEE Transactions on Pattern Analysis and Machine Intelligence* 2001:23, 257–267.

14. MALLAT S. *A Wavelet Tour of Signal Processing*. Academic Press, New York, 1998.

15. SIMONCELLI EP, FREEMAN WT, ADELSON EH, HEEGER DJ. Shiftable multiscale transform. *IEEE Transactions on Information Theory* 1992:38, 587–607.

16. KHONTAZAD A, HONG YH. Invariant image recognition by Zernike moments. *IEEE Transactions on Pattern Analysis and Machine Intelligence* 1990:12, 489–497.

17. TEAGUE MR. Image analysis via the general theory of moments. *Journal of the Optical Society of America* 1980:70, 920–930.

18. TEH CH, CHIN RT. On image analysis by the methods of moments. *IEEE Transactions on Pattern Analysis and Machine Intelligence* 1988:10, 496–513.

19. YAU WC, KUMAR DK, WEGHORN H. Motion features for visual speech recognition. In *Visual Speech Recognition: Lip Segmentation and Mapping*, edited by A Liew, S Wang, 388–415. Medical Information Science Reference, Hershey, PA, 2009.

20. LAPATKI G, STEGEMAN DF, JONAS IE. A surface EMG electrode for the simultaneous observation of multiple facial muscles. *Journal of Neuroscience Methods* 2003:123, 117–128.

21. PARSONS TW. *Voice and Speech Processing,* 1st Edition. McGraw-Hill Book Company, New York, 1986.

22. BASMAJIAN JV, DELUCA CJ. *Muscles Alive: Their Functions Revealed by Electromyography,* 5th Edition. Williams & Wilkins, Baltimore, 1985.

23. CHAN DC, ENGLEHART K, HUDGINS B, LOVELY DF. A multi-expert speech recognition system using acoustic and myoelectric signals. In *Proceedings of the 24th Annual IEEE EMBS/BMES Conference* 2002:1, 72–72.

24. KUMAR S, KUMAR DK, ALEMU M, BURRY M. EMG based voice recognition. In *Proceedings of Intelligent Sensors, Sensor Networks and Information Processing Conference* 2004: 593–597.

25. ARJUNAN SP, KUMAR DK, WEGHORN H, NAIK G. Facial muscle activity patterns for recognition of utterances in native and foreign language: Testing for its reliability and flexibility. In *Cross-Disciplinary Applications of Artificial Intelligence and Pattern Recognition: Advancing Technologies,* edited by V Mago, N Bhatia, 212–231. IGI Global, Hershey, PA, 2012.

26. FOO SW, DONG L. Recognition of Visual Speech Elements Using Hidden Markov Models. *Lecture Notes in Computer Science* 2002: 2532, 607–614.

27. FRIDLUND AJ, CACIOPPO JT. Guidelines for human electromyographic research. *Journal of Biological Psychology* 1986:23(5), 567–589.

28. ARJUNAN SP, YAU WC, KUMAR DK. Evaluating video and facial muscle activity for a better assistive technology: A silent speech based HCI, computational models of complex systems. *Intelligent Systems Reference Library* 2013:53, 89–104.

29. YAU WC. Video analysis of mouth movement using motion templates for computer-based lip-reading. Doctoral dissertation, RMIT University, Melbourne, Australia, 2008. Retrieved from https://researchbank.rmit.edu.au/view/rmit:6864/Yau.pdf. Accessed July 7, 2015.

30. FREEDMAN D, PISANI R, PURVES R. *Statistics.* Norton College Books, New York, 1997.

Index

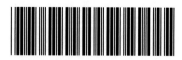